Personal De

Name: ....

Address: ....

....

Email: ....

Mobile Number: ....

Home Number: ....

Emergency Contact

Name: ....

Address: ....

....

Email: ....

Mobile Number: ....

Home Number: ....

Relationship: ....

....

....

Keeping a Fibromyalgia Log

Understanding your pain is a way to beat it. And journaling even a few minutes a day about your chronic pain can be your most powerful tool in decoding the triggers of your pain and mood. And there lies your strength.

If you're a fibromyalgia sufferer, you know that many things can affect your pain. Some of the factors include stress, sleep, daily activities and even the weather. If/When you understand what contributes to your pain level daily, you can begin to work on ways to reduce those pain triggers.

Your knowledge about how your body reacts to those daily triggers can help you to be more in control. And being in more control can eventually help you better manage the pain fibromyalgia brings to your life.

With chronic pain of the fibromyalgia, there comes a lot of stress. Under such strenuous circumstances, keeping track of your symptoms on this journal could help you better pinpoint the causes of your pain and discuss the most successful treatment options with your physicians.

Power of Observation

Fibromyalgia can manifest itself as collection of uncomfortable symptoms. These symptoms can include burning, aching, pulsing or stabbing sensations in any part of the body, and most importantly as musculoskeletal pain.

Through observation of your symptoms and triggers during the day, you can easily highlight trends and track the effectiveness of your current treatments. Sharing these details with your healthcare team can drastically improve your chronic pain management.

Instead of needing to mentally recall how often you have felt pain or how severe it was, you can easily refer to your journal for a detailed record and description.

How to Use This Journal

This journal is designed for simplicity. Because we understand that many people with fibromyalgia or any type of chronic disorders are hesitant to start a pain journal because they think it will take too much of their time.

You don't have to document every moment you experience pain. With the help of easy tracking system this journal offers, you can simply circle the severity of symptoms, or how you feel on the mood scale and add your daily medication and/or supplement details within a few minutes.

Designed by our team member who also has been suffering from fibromyalgia, every bit of graph, and symptom tracker in this journal was carefully curated for ease of use.

You'll be able to track daily:
- The overall level of pain,
- Locations of pain,
- Interference of pain on your sleep,
- The effect of weather changes on your pain,
- Your fatigue during the day,
- Your mood,
- Exercise level,
- Medications and/or supplements.

You'll also have a section for your notes so that you can add additional triggers, water intake, pain patterns that you've noticed as well as your body's reactions to certain food groups.

Each day consists of 2-pages of trackers. They are not pre-dated so that you can use whenever needed.

Stick With It!

Research shows a pain tracking journal is useful when used consistently. The good news is you don't need much time to do it. You can do it when you take your medications, after dinner or before going to bed so that you'd tie that habit to another habit of yours. That will make things easier.

Don't be hard on yourself if you miss a day or two. It'll be okay. Just pick it up and start where you've left.

This will be a life changer for you, your doctors, caregivers, and family.

And last but not least, don't forget: **You got this!**

ZuZu Press Creative Team 🖤

Month: _____ Day: Mon   Tue   Wed   Thu   Fri   Sat   Sun

Overall Level of Pain

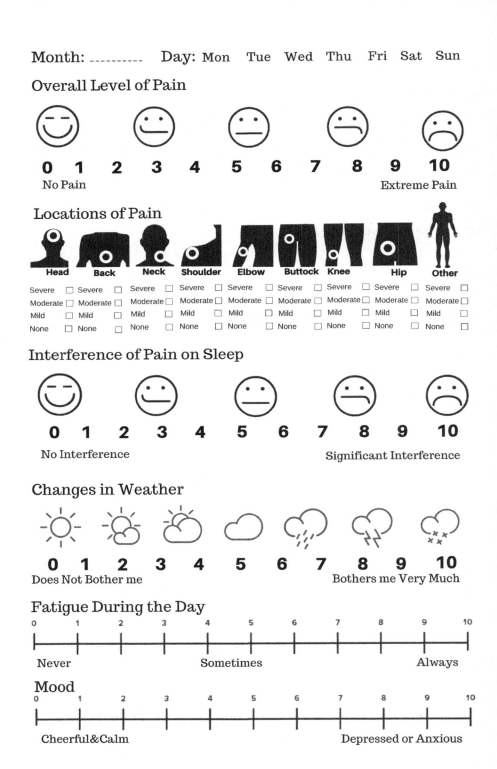

0   1   2   3   4   5   6   7   8   9   10

No Pain   Extreme Pain

Locations of Pain

Head **Back** **Neck** **Shoulder** **Elbow** **Buttock** **Knee** **Hip** **Other**

Head	Back	Neck	Shoulder	Elbow	Buttock	Knee	Hip	Other
Severe ☐	Severe ☐	Severe ☐	Severe ☐	Severe ☐	Severe ☐	Severe ☐	Severe ☐	Severe ☐
Moderate ☐	Moderate ☐	Moderate ☐	Moderate ☐	Moderate ☐	Moderate ☐	Moderate ☐	Moderate ☐	Moderate ☐
Mild ☐	Mild ☐	Mild ☐	Mild ☐	Mild ☐	Mild ☐	Mild ☐	Mild ☐	Mild ☐
None ☐	None ☐	None ☐	None ☐	None ☐	None ☐	None ☐	None ☐	None ☐

Interference of Pain on Sleep

0   1   2   3   4   5   6   7   8   9   10

No Interference   Significant Interference

Changes in Weather

0   1   2   3   4   5   6   7   8   9   10

Does Not Bother me   Bothers me Very Much

Fatigue During the Day

0   1   2   3   4   5   6   7   8   9   10

Never   Sometimes   Always

Mood

0   1   2   3   4   5   6   7   8   9   10

Cheerful&Calm   Depressed or Anxious

Exercise

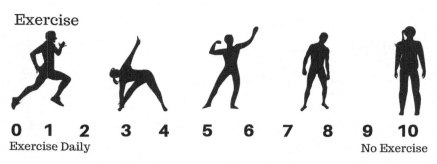

0 1 2 3 4 5 6 7 8 9 10

Exercise Daily   No Exercise

Drugs/Medication

QTY		DESCRIPTION
AM	PM	

Vitamins/Supplements

QTY		DESCRIPTION
AM	PM	

N O T E S

Month: _____ **Day:** Mon Tue Wed Thu Fri Sat Sun

Overall Level of Pain

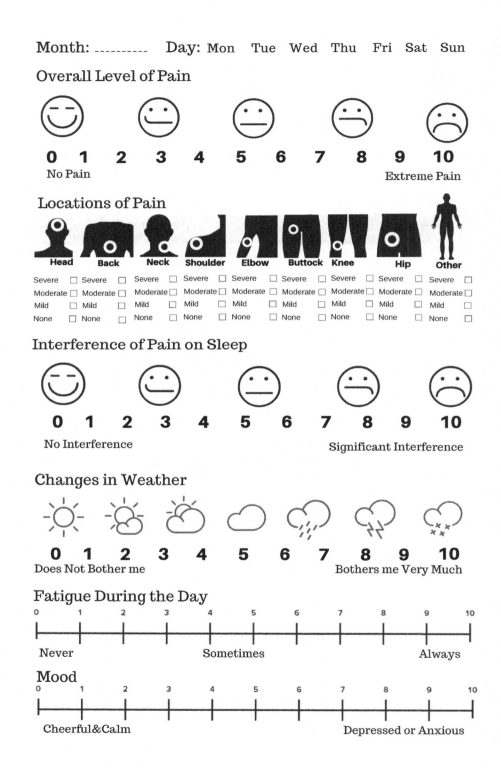

0 1 2 3 4 5 6 7 8 9 10

No Pain   Extreme Pain

Locations of Pain

Head	Back	Neck	Shoulder	Elbow	Buttock	Knee	Hip	Other
Severe ☐	Severe ☐	Severe ☐	Severe ☐	Severe ☐	Severe ☐	Severe ☐	Severe ☐	Severe ☐
Moderate ☐	Moderate ☐	Moderate ☐	Moderate ☐	Moderate ☐	Moderate ☐	Moderate ☐	Moderate ☐	Moderate ☐
Mild ☐	Mild ☐	Mild ☐	Mild ☐	Mild ☐	Mild ☐	Mild ☐	Mild ☐	Mild ☐
None ☐	None ☐	None ☐	None ☐	None ☐	None ☐	None ☐	None ☐	None ☐

Interference of Pain on Sleep

0 1 2 3 4 5 6 7 8 9 10

No Interference   Significant Interference

Changes in Weather

0 1 2 3 4 5 6 7 8 9 10

Does Not Bother me   Bothers me Very Much

Fatigue During the Day

0   1   2   3   4   5   6   7   8   9   10

Never   Sometimes   Always

Mood

0   1   2   3   4   5   6   7   8   9   10

Cheerful&Calm   Depressed or Anxious

Exercise

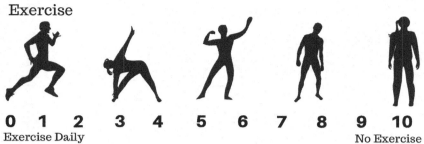

0 1 2 3 4 5 6 7 8 9 10

Exercise Daily   No Exercise

Drugs/Medication

QTY		DESCRIPTION
AM	PM	

Vitamins/Supplements

QTY		DESCRIPTION
AM	PM	

N O T E S

Month: _____ **Day:** Mon   Tue   Wed   Thu   Fri   Sat   Sun

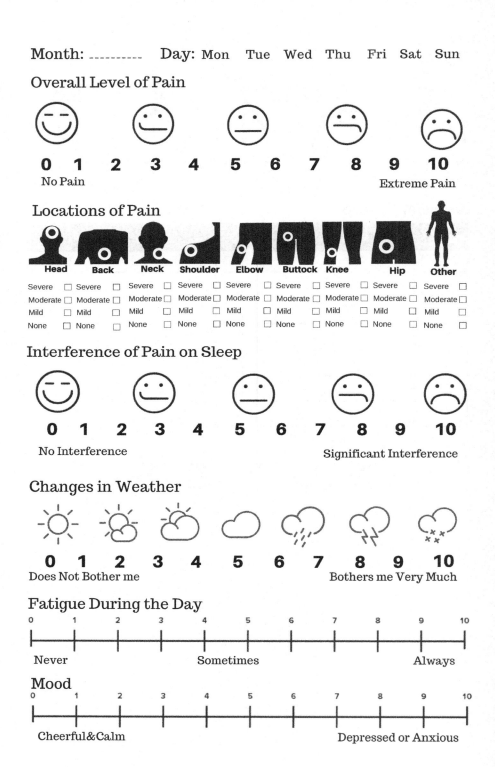

Overall Level of Pain

0   1   2   3   4   5   6   7   8   9   10

No Pain   Extreme Pain

Locations of Pain

Head   Back   Neck   Shoulder   Elbow   Buttock   Knee   Hip   Other

Severe ☐	Severe ☐	Severe ☐	Severe ☐	Severe ☐	Severe ☐	Severe ☐	Severe ☐	Severe ☐
Moderate ☐	Moderate ☐	Moderate ☐	Moderate ☐	Moderate ☐	Moderate ☐	Moderate ☐	Moderate ☐	Moderate ☐
Mild ☐	Mild ☐	Mild ☐	Mild ☐	Mild ☐	Mild ☐	Mild ☐	Mild ☐	Mild ☐
None ☐	None ☐	None ☐	None ☐	None ☐	None ☐	None ☐	None ☐	None ☐

Interference of Pain on Sleep

0   1   2   3   4   5   6   7   8   9   10

No Interference   Significant Interference

Changes in Weather

0   1   2   3   4   5   6   7   8   9   10

Does Not Bother me   Bothers me Very Much

Fatigue During the Day

0   1   2   3   4   5   6   7   8   9   10

Never   Sometimes   Always

Mood

0   1   2   3   4   5   6   7   8   9   10

Cheerful&Calm   Depressed or Anxious

Exercise

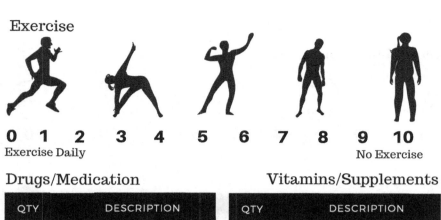

0 1 2 3 4 5 6 7 8 9 10

Exercise Daily   No Exercise

Drugs/Medication

QTY		DESCRIPTION
AM	PM	

Vitamins/Supplements

QTY		DESCRIPTION
AM	PM	

N O T E S

Month: ---------- **Day:** Mon   Tue   Wed   Thu   Fri   Sat   Sun

Overall Level of Pain

0   1   2   3   4   5   6   7   8   9   10

No Pain   Extreme Pain

Locations of Pain

Head	Back	Neck	Shoulder	Elbow	Buttock	Knee	Hip	Other
Severe ☐	Severe ☐	Severe ☐	Severe ☐	Severe ☐	Severe ☐	Severe ☐	Severe ☐	Severe ☐
Moderate ☐	Moderate ☐	Moderate ☐	Moderate ☐	Moderate ☐	Moderate ☐	Moderate ☐	Moderate ☐	Moderate ☐
Mild ☐	Mild ☐	Mild ☐	Mild ☐	Mild ☐	Mild ☐	Mild ☐	Mild ☐	Mild ☐
None ☐	None ☐	None ☐	None ☐	None ☐	None ☐	None ☐	None ☐	None ☐

Interference of Pain on Sleep

0   1   2   3   4   5   6   7   8   9   10

No Interference   Significant Interference

Changes in Weather

0   1   2   3   4   5   6   7   8   9   10

Does Not Bother me   Bothers me Very Much

Fatigue During the Day

0   1   2   3   4   5   6   7   8   9   10

Never   Sometimes   Always

Mood

0   1   2   3   4   5   6   7   8   9   10

Cheerful&Calm   Depressed or Anxious

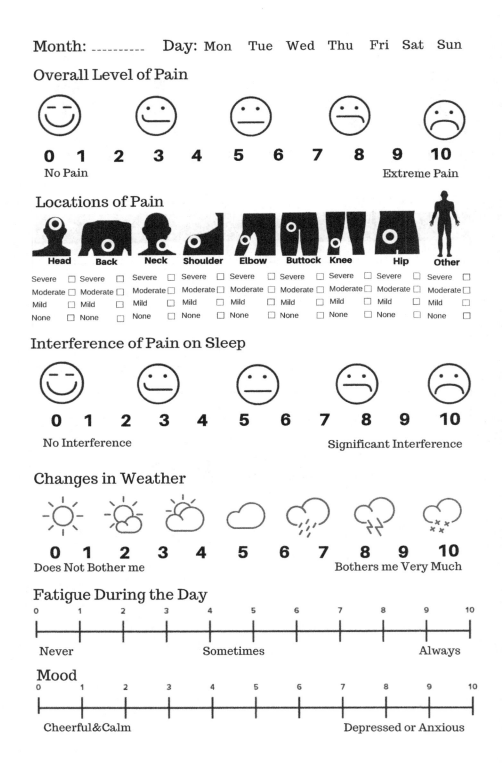

Exercise

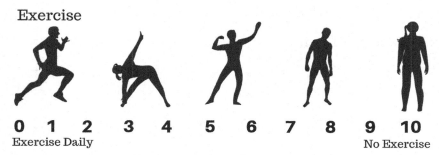

0 1 2   3   4   5   6   7   8   9   10

Exercise Daily   No Exercise

Drugs/Medication

QTY		DESCRIPTION
AM	PM	

Vitamins/Supplements

QTY		DESCRIPTION
AM	PM	

N O T E S

Month: .... **Day:** Mon Tue Wed Thu Fri Sat Sun

Overall Level of Pain

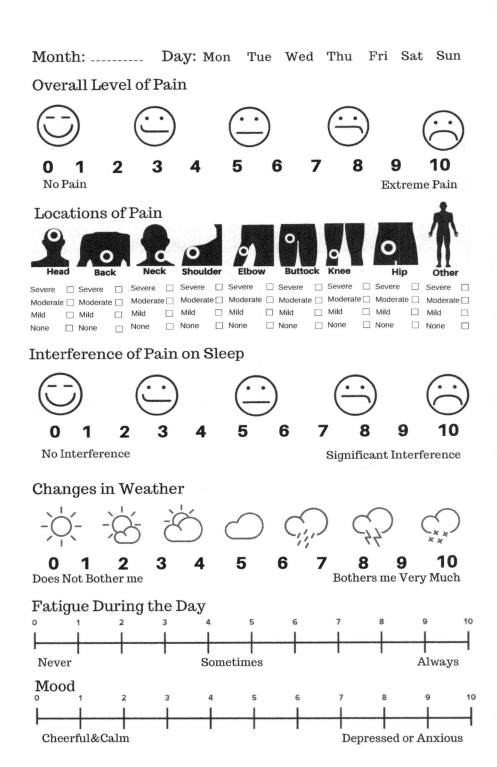

0 1 2 3 4 5 6 7 8 9 10

No Pain   Extreme Pain

Locations of Pain

Head	Back	Neck	Shoulder	Elbow	Buttock	Knee	Hip	Other
Severe ☐	Severe ☐	Severe ☐	Severe ☐	Severe ☐	Severe ☐	Severe ☐	Severe ☐	Severe ☐
Moderate ☐	Moderate ☐	Moderate ☐	Moderate ☐	Moderate ☐	Moderate ☐	Moderate ☐	Moderate ☐	Moderate ☐
Mild ☐	Mild ☐	Mild ☐	Mild ☐	Mild ☐	Mild ☐	Mild ☐	Mild ☐	Mild ☐
None ☐	None ☐	None ☐	None ☐	None ☐	None ☐	None ☐	None ☐	None ☐

Interference of Pain on Sleep

0 1 2 3 4 5 6 7 8 9 10

No Interference   Significant Interference

Changes in Weather

0 1 2 3 4 5 6 7 8 9 10

Does Not Bother me   Bothers me Very Much

Fatigue During the Day

0   1   2   3   4   5   6   7   8   9   10

Never   Sometimes   Always

Mood

0   1   2   3   4   5   6   7   8   9   10

Cheerful&Calm   Depressed or Anxious

Exercise

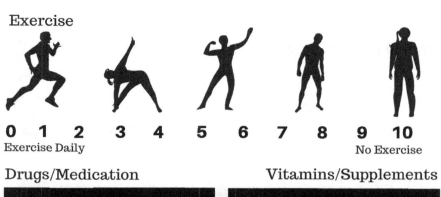

0 1 2 3 4 5 6 7 8 9 10

Exercise Daily   No Exercise

Drugs/Medication

QTY		DESCRIPTION
AM	PM	

Vitamins/Supplements

QTY		DESCRIPTION
AM	PM	

N O T E S

Month: _____ **Day:** Mon Tue Wed Thu Fri Sat Sun

Overall Level of Pain

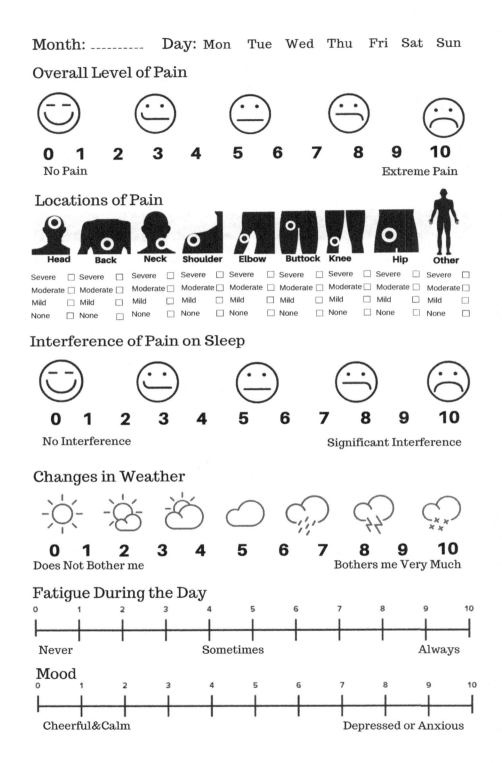

0 1 2 3 4 5 6 7 8 9 10

No Pain   Extreme Pain

Locations of Pain

Head Back Neck Shoulder Elbow Buttock Knee Hip Other

	Head	Back	Neck	Shoulder	Elbow	Buttock	Knee	Hip	Other
Severe	☐	☐	☐	☐	☐	☐	☐	☐	☐
Moderate	☐	☐	☐	☐	☐	☐	☐	☐	☐
Mild	☐	☐	☐	☐	☐	☐	☐	☐	☐
None	☐	☐	☐	☐	☐	☐	☐	☐	☐

Interference of Pain on Sleep

0 1 2 3 4 5 6 7 8 9 10

No Interference   Significant Interference

Changes in Weather

0 1 2 3 4 5 6 7 8 9 10

Does Not Bother me   Bothers me Very Much

Fatigue During the Day

0 1 2 3 4 5 6 7 8 9 10

Never   Sometimes   Always

Mood

0 1 2 3 4 5 6 7 8 9 10

Cheerful&Calm   Depressed or Anxious

Exercise

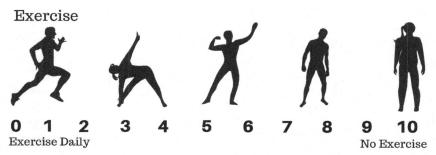

| 0 | 1 | 2 | 3 | 4 | 5 | 6 | 7 | 8 | 9 | 10 |

Exercise Daily   No Exercise

Drugs/Medication

QTY		DESCRIPTION
AM	PM	

Vitamins/Supplements

QTY		DESCRIPTION
AM	PM	

N O T E S

Month: _____ Day: Mon Tue Wed Thu Fri Sat Sun

Overall Level of Pain

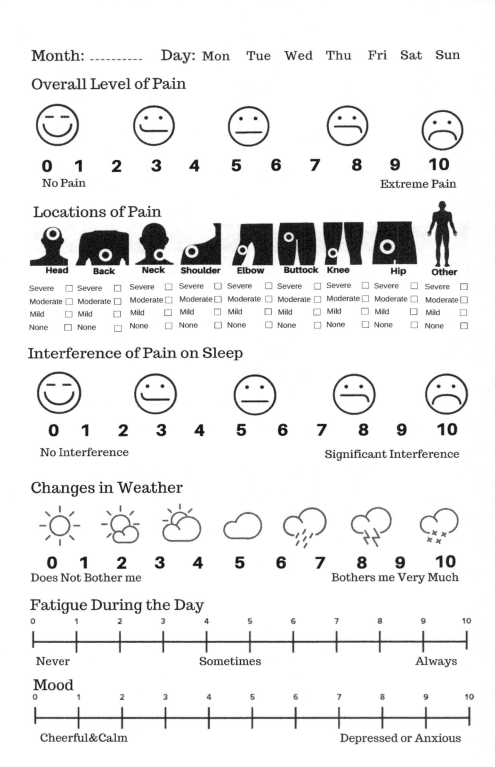

0 1 2 3 4 5 6 7 8 9 10
No Pain   Extreme Pain

Locations of Pain

	Head	Back	Neck	Shoulder	Elbow	Buttock	Knee	Hip	Other
Severe	☐	☐	☐	☐	☐	☐	☐	☐	☐
Moderate	☐	☐	☐	☐	☐	☐	☐	☐	☐
Mild	☐	☐	☐	☐	☐	☐	☐	☐	☐
None	☐	☐	☐	☐	☐	☐	☐	☐	☐

Interference of Pain on Sleep

0 1 2 3 4 5 6 7 8 9 10
No Interference   Significant Interference

Changes in Weather

0 1 2 3 4 5 6 7 8 9 10
Does Not Bother me   Bothers me Very Much

Fatigue During the Day

0   1   2   3   4   5   6   7   8   9   10
Never   Sometimes   Always

Mood

0   1   2   3   4   5   6   7   8   9   10
Cheerful&Calm   Depressed or Anxious

Exercise

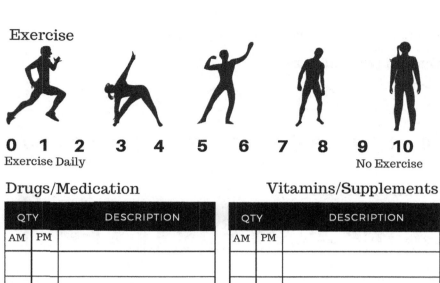

0   1   2   3   4   5   6   7   8   9   10

Exercise Daily   No Exercise

Drugs/Medication

QTY		DESCRIPTION
AM	PM	

Vitamins/Supplements

QTY		DESCRIPTION
AM	PM	

N O T E S

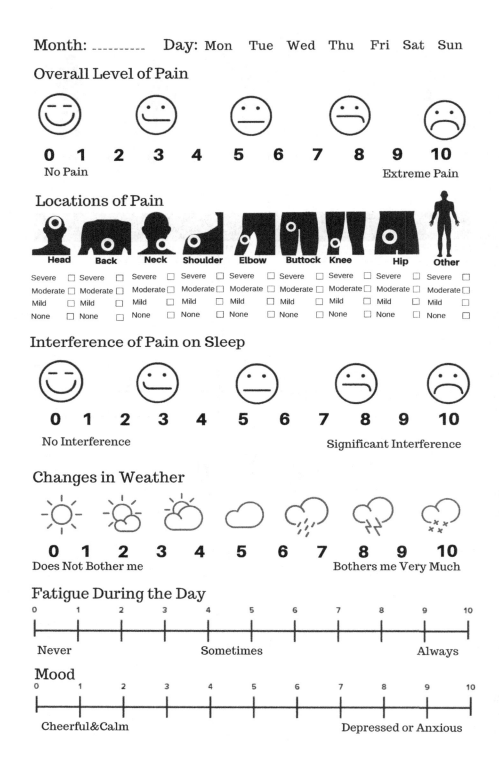

Month: .... **Day:** Mon Tue Wed Thu Fri Sat Sun

Overall Level of Pain

0   1   2   3   4   5   6   7   8   9   10

No Pain   Extreme Pain

Locations of Pain

	Head	Back	Neck	Shoulder	Elbow	Buttock	Knee	Hip	Other
Severe	☐	☐	☐	☐	☐	☐	☐	☐	☐
Moderate	☐	☐	☐	☐	☐	☐	☐	☐	☐
Mild	☐	☐	☐	☐	☐	☐	☐	☐	☐
None	☐	☐	☐	☐	☐	☐	☐	☐	☐

Interference of Pain on Sleep

0   1   2   3   4   5   6   7   8   9   10

No Interference   Significant Interference

Changes in Weather

0   1   2   3   4   5   6   7   8   9   10

Does Not Bother me   Bothers me Very Much

Fatigue During the Day

0   1   2   3   4   5   6   7   8   9   10

Never   Sometimes   Always

Mood

0   1   2   3   4   5   6   7   8   9   10

Cheerful&Calm   Depressed or Anxious

Exercise

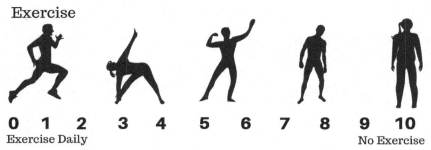

0 1 2   3   4   5   6   7   8   9 10

Exercise Daily   No Exercise

Drugs/Medication

QTY		DESCRIPTION
AM	PM	

Vitamins/Supplements

QTY		DESCRIPTION
AM	PM	

N O T E S

Month: _____ **Day:** Mon Tue Wed Thu Fri Sat Sun

Overall Level of Pain

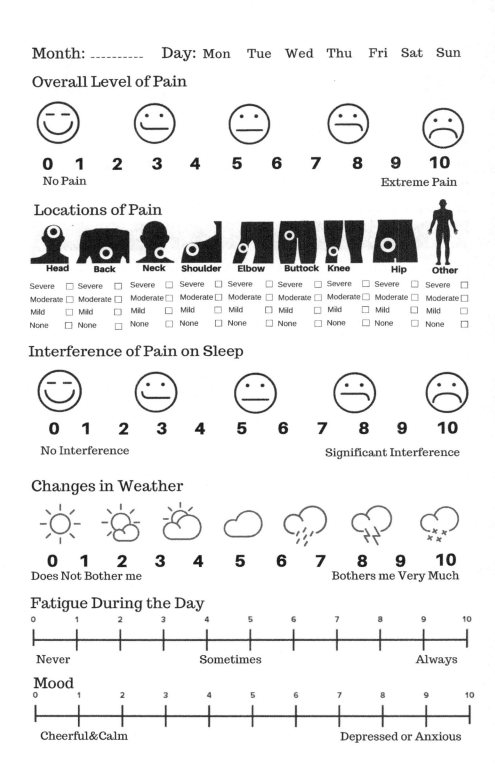

0 1 2 3 4 5 6 7 8 9 10

No Pain   Extreme Pain

Locations of Pain

	Head	Back	Neck	Shoulder	Elbow	Buttock	Knee	Hip	Other
Severe	☐	☐	☐	☐	☐	☐	☐	☐	☐
Moderate	☐	☐	☐	☐	☐	☐	☐	☐	☐
Mild	☐	☐	☐	☐	☐	☐	☐	☐	☐
None	☐	☐	☐	☐	☐	☐	☐	☐	☐

Interference of Pain on Sleep

0 1 2 3 4 5 6 7 8 9 10

No Interference   Significant Interference

Changes in Weather

0 1 2 3 4 5 6 7 8 9 10

Does Not Bother me   Bothers me Very Much

Fatigue During the Day

0   1   2   3   4   5   6   7   8   9   10

Never   Sometimes   Always

Mood

0   1   2   3   4   5   6   7   8   9   10

Cheerful&Calm   Depressed or Anxious

Exercise

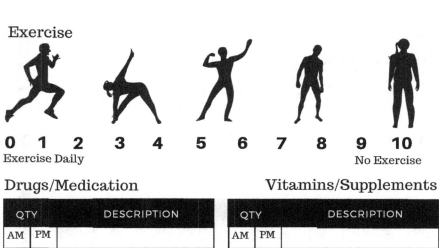

| 0 | 1 | 2 | 3 | 4 | 5 | 6 | 7 | 8 | 9 | 10 |

Exercise Daily   **No Exercise**

Drugs/Medication

QTY		DESCRIPTION
AM	PM	

Vitamins/Supplements

QTY		DESCRIPTION
AM	PM	

N O T E S

Month: ---------- **Day:** Mon   Tue   Wed   Thu   Fri   Sat   Sun

Overall Level of Pain

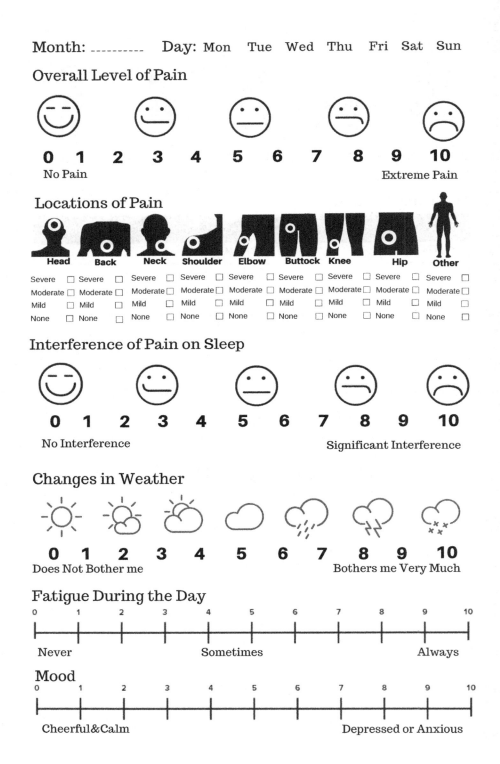

0   1   2   3   4   5   6   7   8   9   10

No Pain   Extreme Pain

Locations of Pain

	Head	Back	Neck	Shoulder	Elbow	Buttock	Knee	Hip	Other
Severe	☐	☐	☐	☐	☐	☐	☐	☐	☐
Moderate	☐	☐	☐	☐	☐	☐	☐	☐	☐
Mild	☐	☐	☐	☐	☐	☐	☐	☐	☐
None	☐	☐	☐	☐	☐	☐	☐	☐	☐

Interference of Pain on Sleep

0   1   2   3   4   5   6   7   8   9   10

No Interference   Significant Interference

Changes in Weather

0   1   2   3   4   5   6   7   8   9   10

Does Not Bother me   Bothers me Very Much

Fatigue During the Day

0   1   2   3   4   5   6   7   8   9   10

Never   Sometimes   Always

Mood

0   1   2   3   4   5   6   7   8   9   10

Cheerful&Calm   Depressed or Anxious

Exercise

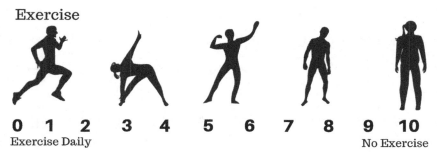

0 1 2   3   4   5   6   7   8   9   10

Exercise Daily   No Exercise

Drugs/Medication

QTY		DESCRIPTION
AM	PM	

Vitamins/Supplements

QTY		DESCRIPTION
AM	PM	

N O T E S

Month: ---------- **Day:** Mon Tue Wed Thu Fri Sat Sun

Overall Level of Pain

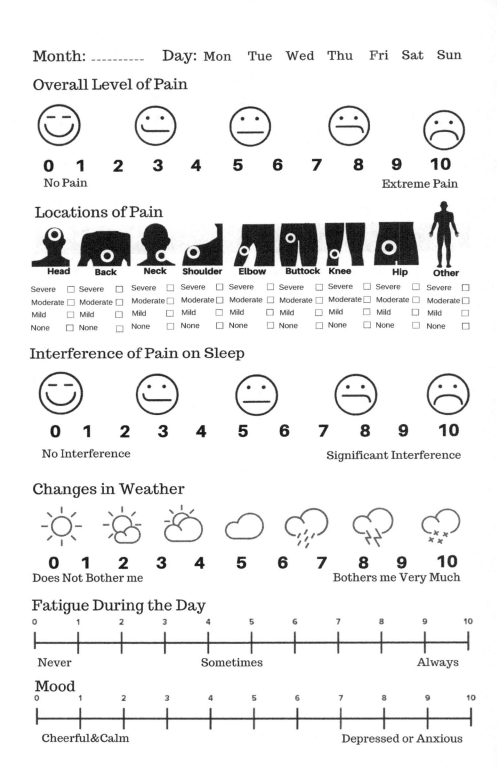

0 1 2 3 4 5 6 7 8 9 10

No Pain

Extreme Pain

Locations of Pain

	Head	Back	Neck	Shoulder	Elbow	Buttock	Knee	Hip	Other
Severe	☐	☐	☐	☐	☐	☐	☐	☐	☐
Moderate	☐	☐	☐	☐	☐	☐	☐	☐	☐
Mild	☐	☐	☐	☐	☐	☐	☐	☐	☐
None	☐	☐	☐	☐	☐	☐	☐	☐	☐

Interference of Pain on Sleep

0 1 2 3 4 5 6 7 8 9 10

No Interference

Significant Interference

Changes in Weather

0 1 2 3 4 5 6 7 8 9 10

Does Not Bother me

Bothers me Very Much

Fatigue During the Day

0   1   2   3   4   5   6   7   8   9   10

Never   Sometimes   Always

Mood

0   1   2   3   4   5   6   7   8   9   10

Cheerful&Calm   Depressed or Anxious

Exercise

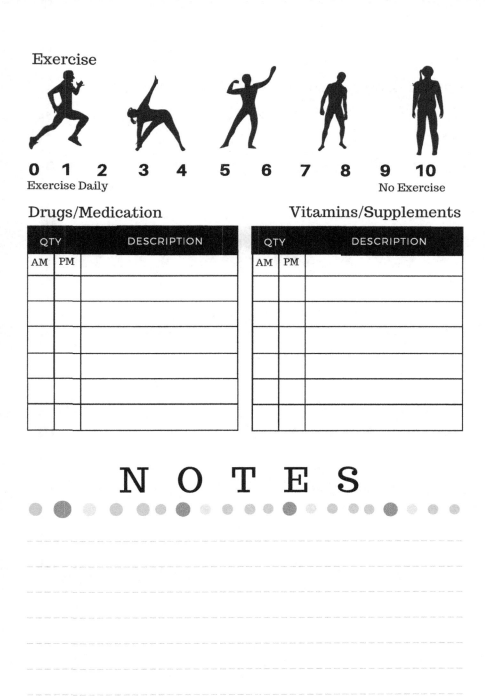

0 1 2 3 4 5 6 7 8 9 10

Exercise Daily   No Exercise

Drugs/Medication

QTY		DESCRIPTION
AM	PM	

Vitamins/Supplements

QTY		DESCRIPTION
AM	PM	

N O T E S

Month: .... **Day:** Mon Tue Wed Thu Fri Sat Sun

Overall Level of Pain

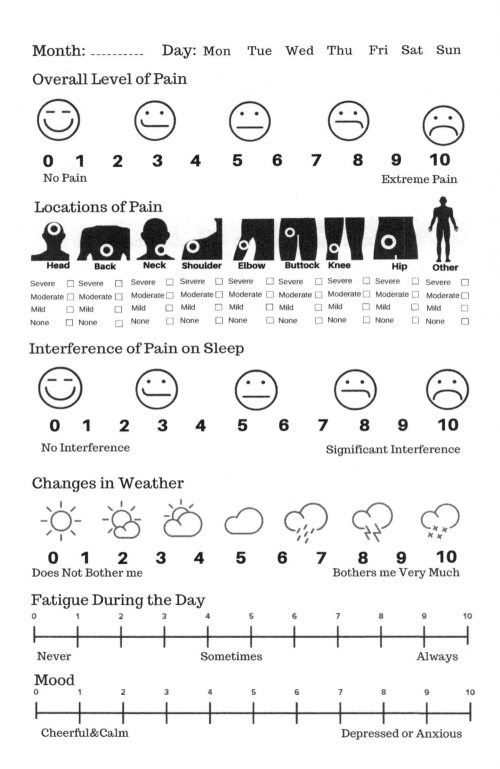

0 1 2 3 4 5 6 7 8 9 10

No Pain

Extreme Pain

Locations of Pain

	Head	Back	Neck	Shoulder	Elbow	Buttock	Knee	Hip	Other
Severe	☐	☐	☐	☐	☐	☐	☐	☐	☐
Moderate	☐	☐	☐	☐	☐	☐	☐	☐	☐
Mild	☐	☐	☐	☐	☐	☐	☐	☐	☐
None	☐	☐	☐	☐	☐	☐	☐	☐	☐

Interference of Pain on Sleep

0 1 2 3 4 5 6 7 8 9 10

No Interference

Significant Interference

Changes in Weather

0 1 2 3 4 5 6 7 8 9 10

Does Not Bother me

Bothers me Very Much

Fatigue During the Day

0 1 2 3 4 5 6 7 8 9 10

Never   Sometimes   Always

Mood

0 1 2 3 4 5 6 7 8 9 10

Cheerful&Calm   Depressed or Anxious

Exercise

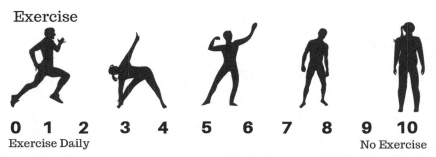

0 1 2   3   4   5   6   7   8   9   10

Exercise Daily   No Exercise

Drugs/Medication

QTY		DESCRIPTION
AM	PM	

Vitamins/Supplements

QTY		DESCRIPTION
AM	PM	

N O T E S

Month: ---------- **Day:** Mon Tue Wed Thu Fri Sat Sun

Overall Level of Pain

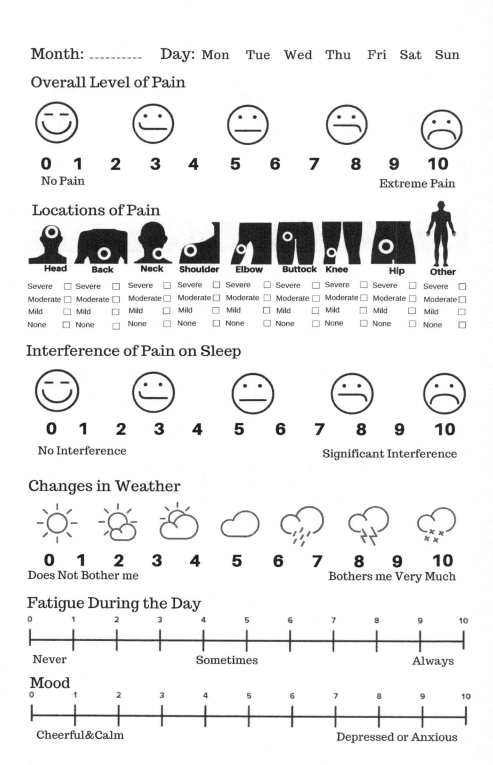

0   1   2   3   4   5   6   7   8   9   10

No Pain   Extreme Pain

Locations of Pain

Head	Back	Neck	Shoulder	Elbow	Buttock	Knee	Hip	Other
Severe ☐	Severe ☐	Severe ☐	Severe ☐	Severe ☐	Severe ☐	Severe ☐	Severe ☐	Severe ☐
Moderate ☐	Moderate ☐	Moderate ☐	Moderate ☐	Moderate ☐	Moderate ☐	Moderate ☐	Moderate ☐	Moderate ☐
Mild ☐	Mild ☐	Mild ☐	Mild ☐	Mild ☐	Mild ☐	Mild ☐	Mild ☐	Mild ☐
None ☐	None ☐	None ☐	None ☐	None ☐	None ☐	None ☐	None ☐	None ☐

Interference of Pain on Sleep

0   1   2   3   4   5   6   7   8   9   10

No Interference   Significant Interference

Changes in Weather

0   1   2   3   4   5   6   7   8   9   10

Does Not Bother me   Bothers me Very Much

Fatigue During the Day

0   1   2   3   4   5   6   7   8   9   10

Never   Sometimes   Always

Mood

0   1   2   3   4   5   6   7   8   9   10

Cheerful&Calm   Depressed or Anxious

Exercise

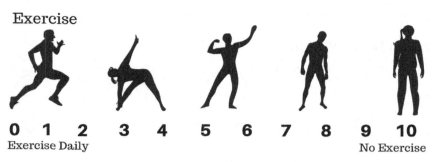

0   1   2   3   4   5   6   7   8   9   10

Exercise Daily   No Exercise

Drugs/Medication

QTY		DESCRIPTION
AM	PM	

Vitamins/Supplements

QTY		DESCRIPTION
AM	PM	

N O T E S

Month: ---------- Day: Mon Tue Wed Thu Fri Sat Sun

Overall Level of Pain

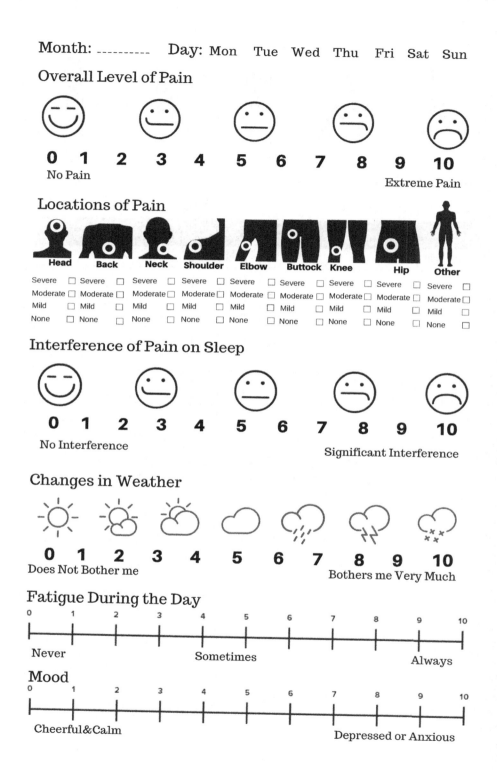

0 1 2 3 4 5 6 7 8 9 10

No Pain

Extreme Pain

Locations of Pain

	Head	Back	Neck	Shoulder	Elbow	Buttock	Knee	Hip	Other
Severe	☐	☐	☐	☐	☐	☐	☐	☐	☐
Moderate	☐	☐	☐	☐	☐	☐	☐	☐	☐
Mild	☐	☐	☐	☐	☐	☐	☐	☐	☐
None	☐	☐	☐	☐	☐	☐	☐	☐	☐

Interference of Pain on Sleep

0 1 2 3 4 5 6 7 8 9 10

No Interference

Significant Interference

Changes in Weather

0 1 2 3 4 5 6 7 8 9 10

Does Not Bother me

Bothers me Very Much

Fatigue During the Day

0 1 2 3 4 5 6 7 8 9 10

Never

Sometimes

Always

Mood

0 1 2 3 4 5 6 7 8 9 10

Cheerful&Calm

Depressed or Anxious

Exercise

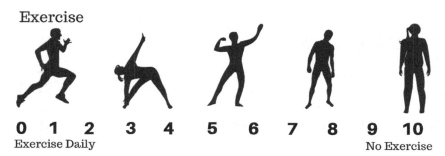

0 1 2 3 4 5 6 7 8 9 10

Exercise Daily   No Exercise

Drugs/Medication

QTY		DESCRIPTION
AM	PM	

Vitamins/Supplements

QTY		DESCRIPTION
AM	PM	

N O T E S

Month: _____ Day: Mon Tue Wed Thu Fri Sat Sun

Overall Level of Pain

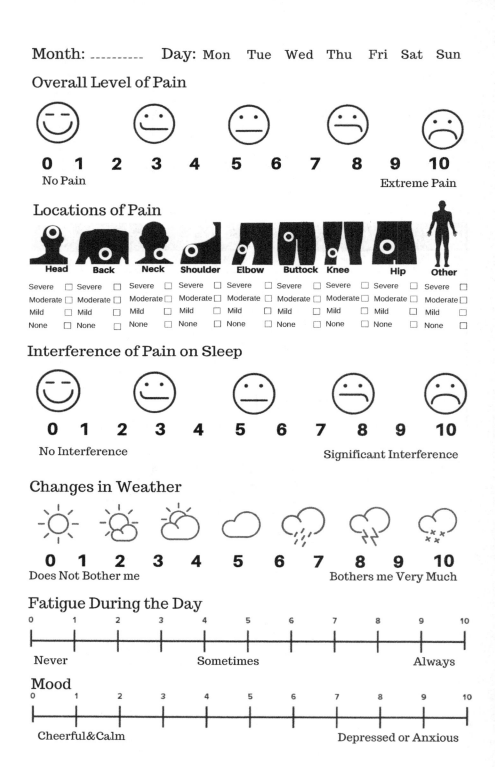

0   1   2   3   4   5   6   7   8   9   10

No Pain   Extreme Pain

Locations of Pain

	Head	Back	Neck	Shoulder	Elbow	Buttock	Knee	Hip	Other
Severe	☐	Severe ☐	Severe ☐	Severe ☐	Severe ☐	Severe ☐	Severe ☐	Severe ☐	Severe ☐
Moderate	☐	Moderate ☐	Moderate ☐	Moderate ☐	Moderate ☐	Moderate ☐	Moderate ☐	Moderate ☐	Moderate ☐
Mild	☐	Mild ☐	Mild ☐	Mild ☐	Mild ☐	Mild ☐	Mild ☐	Mild ☐	Mild ☐
None	☐	None ☐	None ☐	None ☐	None ☐	None ☐	None ☐	None ☐	None ☐

Interference of Pain on Sleep

0   1   2   3   4   5   6   7   8   9   10

No Interference   Significant Interference

Changes in Weather

0   1   2   3   4   5   6   7   8   9   10

Does Not Bother me   Bothers me Very Much

Fatigue During the Day

0   1   2   3   4   5   6   7   8   9   10

Never   Sometimes   Always

Mood

0   1   2   3   4   5   6   7   8   9   10

Cheerful&Calm   Depressed or Anxious

Exercise

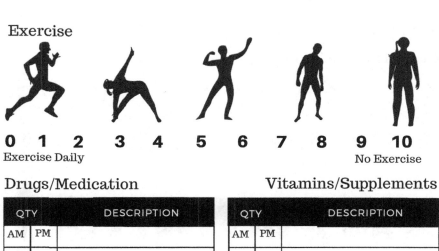

0   1   2   3   4   5   6   7   8   9   10

Exercise Daily   No Exercise

Drugs/Medication

QTY		DESCRIPTION
AM	PM	

Vitamins/Supplements

QTY		DESCRIPTION
AM	PM	

N O T E S

Month: ---------- **Day:** Mon Tue Wed Thu Fri Sat Sun

Overall Level of Pain

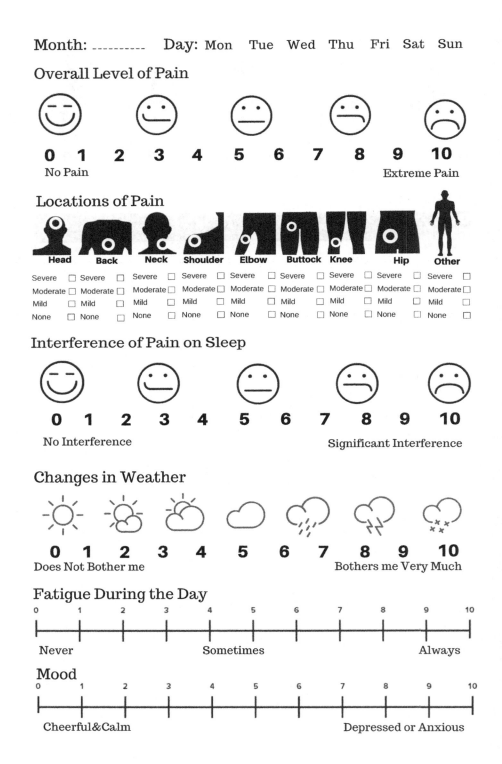

0 1 2 3 4 5 6 7 8 9 10

No Pain   Extreme Pain

Locations of Pain

	Head	Back	Neck	Shoulder	Elbow	Buttock	Knee	Hip	Other
Severe	☐	☐	☐	☐	☐	☐	☐	☐	☐
Moderate	☐	☐	☐	☐	☐	☐	☐	☐	☐
Mild	☐	☐	☐	☐	☐	☐	☐	☐	☐
None	☐	☐	☐	☐	☐	☐	☐	☐	☐

Interference of Pain on Sleep

0 1 2 3 4 5 6 7 8 9 10

No Interference   Significant Interference

Changes in Weather

0 1 2 3 4 5 6 7 8 9 10

Does Not Bother me   Bothers me Very Much

Fatigue During the Day

0   1   2   3   4   5   6   7   8   9   10

Never   Sometimes   Always

Mood

0   1   2   3   4   5   6   7   8   9   10

Cheerful&Calm   Depressed or Anxious

Exercise

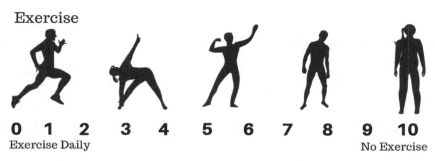

0   1   2   3   4   5   6   7   8   9   10

Exercise Daily   No Exercise

Drugs/Medication

QTY		DESCRIPTION
AM	PM	

Vitamins/Supplements

QTY		DESCRIPTION
AM	PM	

N O T E S

Month: _____ **Day:** Mon Tue Wed Thu Fri Sat Sun

Overall Level of Pain

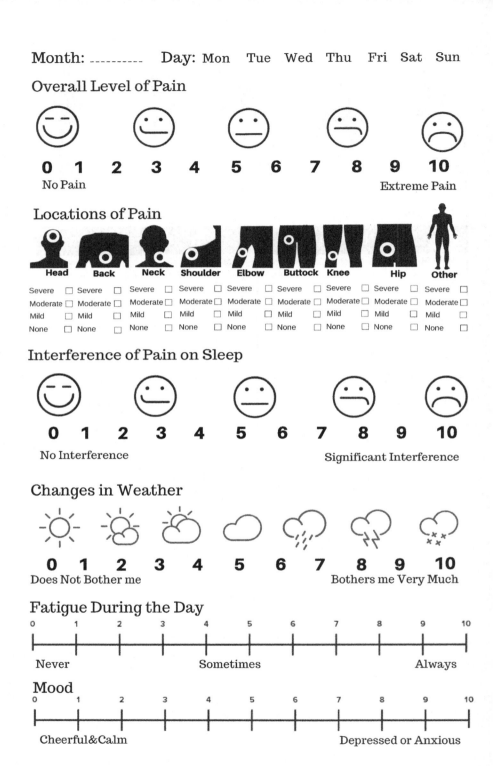

0 1 2 3 4 5 6 7 8 9 10

No Pain   Extreme Pain

Locations of Pain

Head	Back	Neck	Shoulder	Elbow	Buttock	Knee	Hip	Other
Severe ☐	Severe ☐	Severe ☐	Severe ☐	Severe ☐	Severe ☐	Severe ☐	Severe ☐	Severe ☐
Moderate ☐	Moderate ☐	Moderate ☐	Moderate ☐	Moderate ☐	Moderate ☐	Moderate ☐	Moderate ☐	Moderate ☐
Mild ☐	Mild ☐	Mild ☐	Mild ☐	Mild ☐	Mild ☐	Mild ☐	Mild ☐	Mild ☐
None ☐	None ☐	None ☐	None ☐	None ☐	None ☐	None ☐	None ☐	None ☐

Interference of Pain on Sleep

0 1 2 3 4 5 6 7 8 9 10

No Interference   Significant Interference

Changes in Weather

0 1 2 3 4 5 6 7 8 9 10

Does Not Bother me   Bothers me Very Much

Fatigue During the Day

0   1   2   3   4   5   6   7   8   9   10

Never   Sometimes   Always

Mood

0   1   2   3   4   5   6   7   8   9   10

Cheerful&Calm   Depressed or Anxious

Exercise

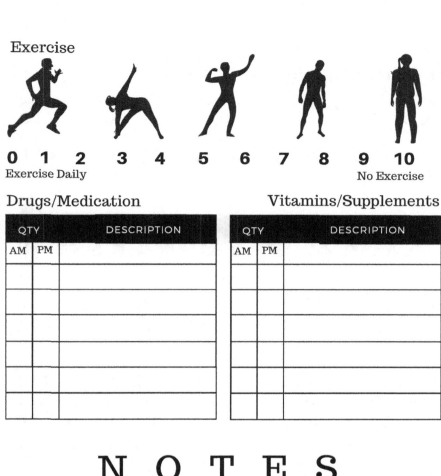

0 1 2 3 4 5 6 7 8 9 10

Exercise Daily No Exercise

Drugs/Medication

QTY		DESCRIPTION
AM	PM	

Vitamins/Supplements

QTY		DESCRIPTION
AM	PM	

N O T E S

Month: ---------- **Day:** Mon Tue Wed Thu Fri Sat Sun

Overall Level of Pain

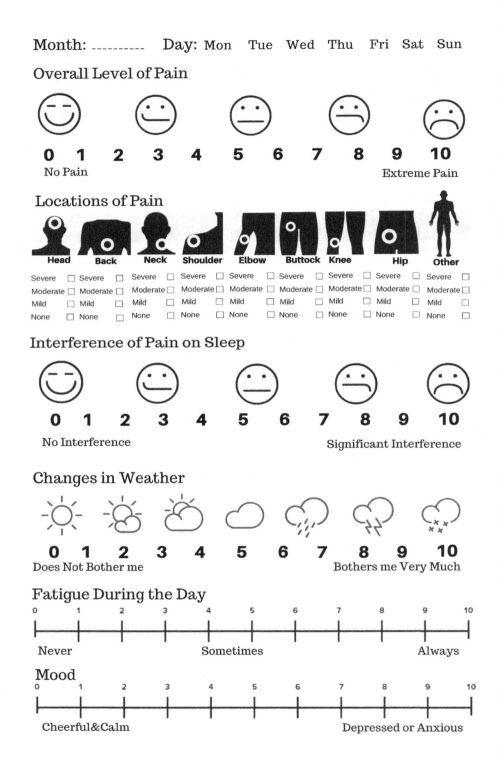

0 1 2 3 4 5 6 7 8 9 10

No Pain   Extreme Pain

Locations of Pain

	Head	Back	Neck	Shoulder	Elbow	Buttock	Knee	Hip	Other
Severe	☐	☐	☐	☐	☐	☐	☐	☐	☐
Moderate	☐	☐	☐	☐	☐	☐	☐	☐	☐
Mild	☐	☐	☐	☐	☐	☐	☐	☐	☐
None	☐	☐	☐	☐	☐	☐	☐	☐	☐

Interference of Pain on Sleep

0 1 2 3 4 5 6 7 8 9 10

No Interference   Significant Interference

Changes in Weather

0 1 2 3 4 5 6 7 8 9 10

Does Not Bother me   Bothers me Very Much

Fatigue During the Day

0 1 2 3 4 5 6 7 8 9 10

Never   Sometimes   Always

Mood

0 1 2 3 4 5 6 7 8 9 10

Cheerful&Calm   Depressed or Anxious

Exercise

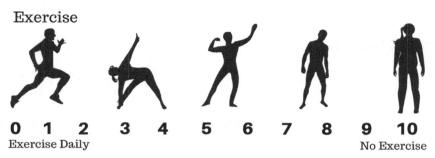

0   1   2   3   4   5   6   7   8   9   10

Exercise Daily   No Exercise

Drugs/Medication

QTY		DESCRIPTION
AM	PM	

Vitamins/Supplements

QTY		DESCRIPTION
AM	PM	

N O T E S

Month: ---------- **Day:** Mon Tue Wed Thu Fri Sat Sun

Overall Level of Pain

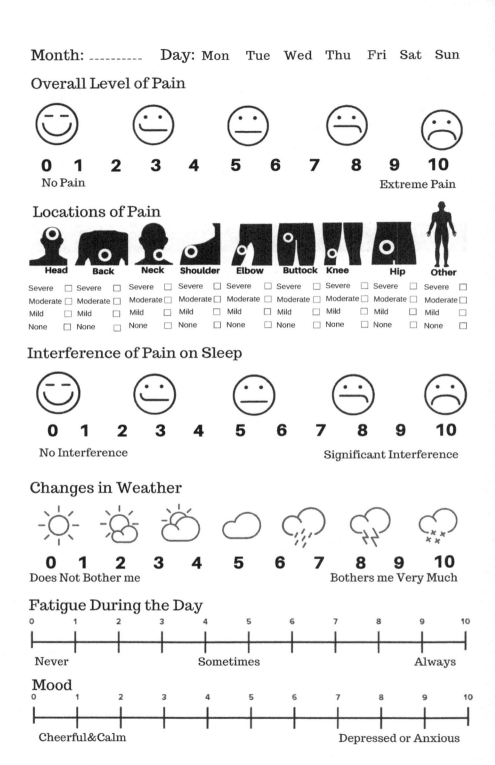

0 1 2 3 4 5 6 7 8 9 10

No Pain   Extreme Pain

Locations of Pain

	Head	Back	Neck	Shoulder	Elbow	Buttock	Knee	Hip	Other
Severe	☐	☐	☐	☐	☐	☐	☐	☐	☐
Moderate	☐	☐	☐	☐	☐	☐	☐	☐	☐
Mild	☐	☐	☐	☐	☐	☐	☐	☐	☐
None	☐	☐	☐	☐	☐	☐	☐	☐	☐

Interference of Pain on Sleep

0 1 2 3 4 5 6 7 8 9 10

No Interference   Significant Interference

Changes in Weather

0 1 2 3 4 5 6 7 8 9 10

Does Not Bother me   Bothers me Very Much

Fatigue During the Day

0 1 2 3 4 5 6 7 8 9 10

Never   Sometimes   Always

Mood

0 1 2 3 4 5 6 7 8 9 10

Cheerful&Calm   Depressed or Anxious

Exercise

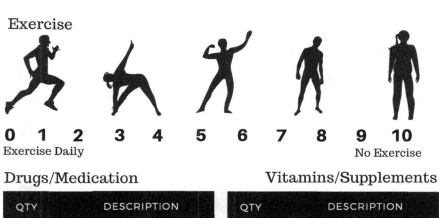

| 0 | 1 | 2 | 3 | 4 | 5 | 6 | 7 | 8 | 9 | 10 |

Exercise Daily   No Exercise

Drugs/Medication

QTY		DESCRIPTION
AM	PM	

Vitamins/Supplements

QTY		DESCRIPTION
AM	PM	

N O T E S

Month: ---------- **Day:** Mon Tue Wed Thu Fri Sat Sun

Overall Level of Pain

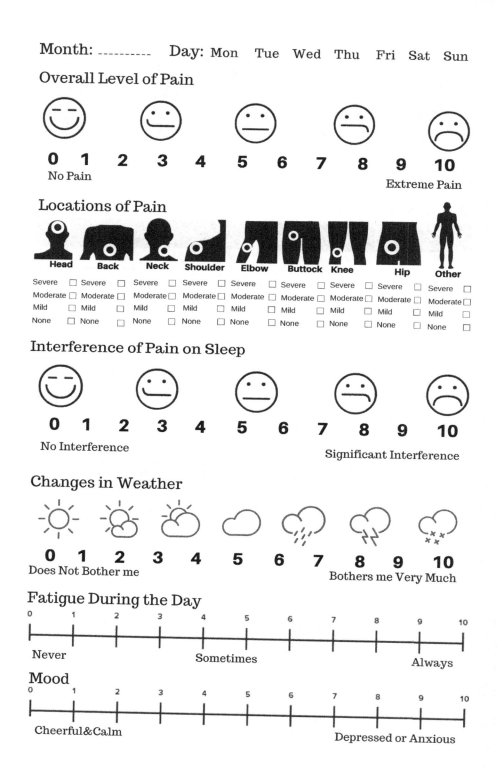

0 1 2 3 4 5 6 7 8 9 10

No Pain

Extreme Pain

Locations of Pain

Head   Back   Neck   Shoulder   Elbow   Buttock   Knee   Hip   Other

	Head	Back	Neck	Shoulder	Elbow	Buttock	Knee	Hip	Other
Severe	☐	☐	☐	☐	☐	☐	☐	☐	☐
Moderate	☐	☐	☐	☐	☐	☐	☐	☐	☐
Mild	☐	☐	☐	☐	☐	☐	☐	☐	☐
None	☐	☐	☐	☐	☐	☐	☐	☐	☐

Interference of Pain on Sleep

0 1 2 3 4 5 6 7 8 9 10

No Interference

Significant Interference

Changes in Weather

0 1 2 3 4 5 6 7 8 9 10

Does Not Bother me

Bothers me Very Much

Fatigue During the Day

0   1   2   3   4   5   6   7   8   9   10

Never   Sometimes   Always

Mood

0   1   2   3   4   5   6   7   8   9   10

Cheerful&Calm   Depressed or Anxious

Exercise

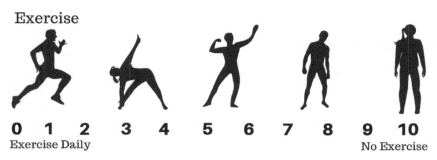

| 0 | 1 | 2 | 3 | 4 | 5 | 6 | 7 | 8 | 9 | 10 |

Exercise Daily   No Exercise

Drugs/Medication

QTY		DESCRIPTION
AM	PM	

Vitamins/Supplements

QTY		DESCRIPTION
AM	PM	

N O T E S

Month: _____ Day: Mon Tue Wed Thu Fri Sat Sun

Overall Level of Pain

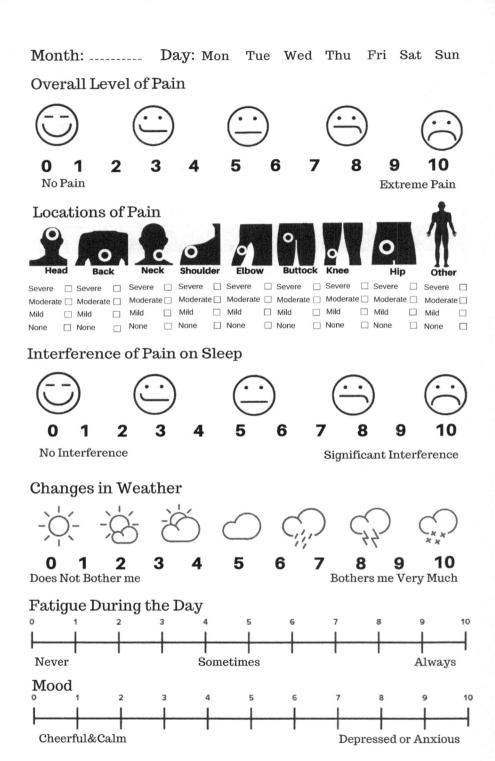

0 1 2 3 4 5 6 7 8 9 10

No Pain   Extreme Pain

Locations of Pain

	Head	Back	Neck	Shoulder	Elbow	Buttock	Knee	Hip	Other
Severe	☐	☐	☐	☐	☐	☐	☐	☐	☐
Moderate	☐	☐	☐	☐	☐	☐	☐	☐	☐
Mild	☐	☐	☐	☐	☐	☐	☐	☐	☐
None	☐	☐	☐	☐	☐	☐	☐	☐	☐

Interference of Pain on Sleep

0 1 2 3 4 5 6 7 8 9 10

No Interference   Significant Interference

Changes in Weather

0 1 2 3 4 5 6 7 8 9 10

Does Not Bother me   Bothers me Very Much

Fatigue During the Day

0   1   2   3   4   5   6   7   8   9   10

Never   Sometimes   Always

Mood

0   1   2   3   4   5   6   7   8   9   10

Cheerful&Calm   Depressed or Anxious

Exercise

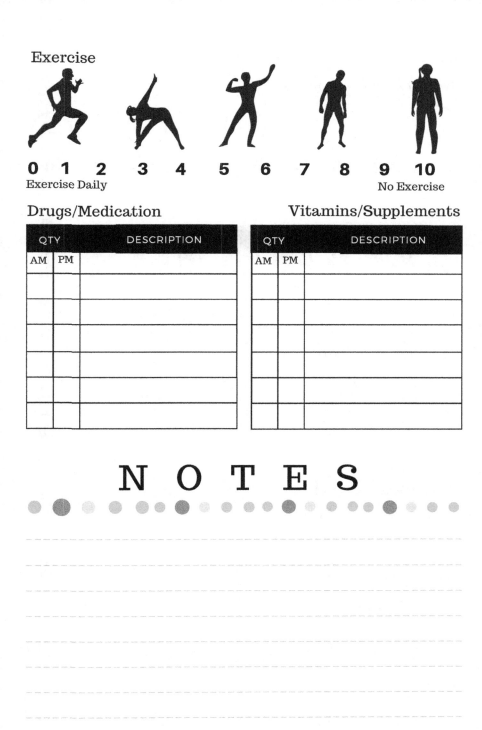

0   1   2   3   4   5   6   7   8   9   10

Exercise Daily   No Exercise

Drugs/Medication

QTY		DESCRIPTION
AM	PM	

Vitamins/Supplements

QTY		DESCRIPTION
AM	PM	

N O T E S

Month: ---------- **Day:** Mon Tue Wed Thu Fri Sat Sun

Overall Level of Pain

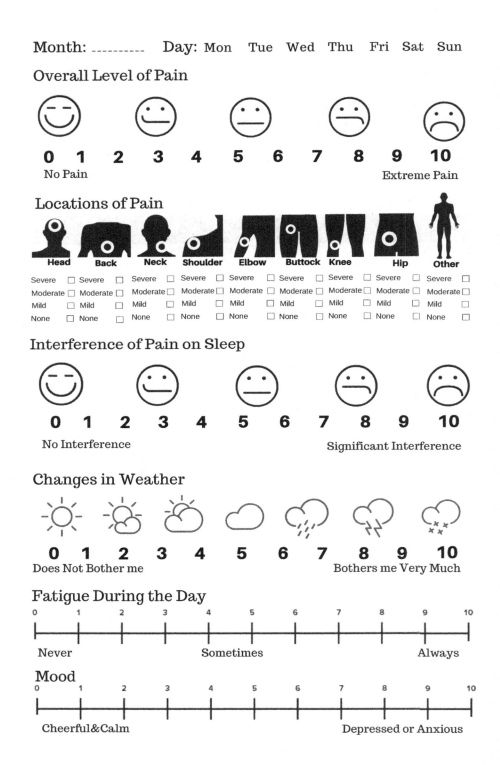

0　1　2　3　4　5　6　7　8　9　10

No Pain　　　　　　　　　　　　　　Extreme Pain

Locations of Pain

	Head	Back	Neck	Shoulder	Elbow	Buttock	Knee	Hip	Other
Severe	☐	☐	☐	☐	☐	☐	☐	☐	☐
Moderate	☐	☐	☐	☐	☐	☐	☐	☐	☐
Mild	☐	☐	☐	☐	☐	☐	☐	☐	☐
None	☐	☐	☐	☐	☐	☐	☐	☐	☐

Interference of Pain on Sleep

0　1　2　3　4　5　6　7　8　9　10

No Interference　　　　　　　Significant Interference

Changes in Weather

0　1　2　3　4　5　6　7　8　9　10

Does Not Bother me　　　　　Bothers me Very Much

Fatigue During the Day

0　1　2　3　4　5　6　7　8　9　10

Never　　　　Sometimes　　　　Always

Mood

0　1　2　3　4　5　6　7　8　9　10

Cheerful&Calm　　　　Depressed or Anxious

Exercise

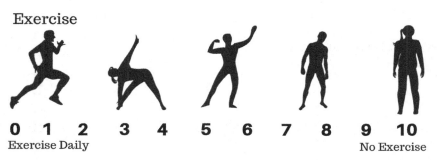

| 0 | 1 | 2 | 3 | 4 | 5 | 6 | 7 | 8 | 9 | 10 |

Exercise Daily   No Exercise

Drugs/Medication

QTY		DESCRIPTION
AM	PM	

Vitamins/Supplements

QTY		DESCRIPTION
AM	PM	

N O T E S

Month: _____ **Day:** Mon　Tue　Wed　Thu　Fri　Sat　Sun

Overall Level of Pain

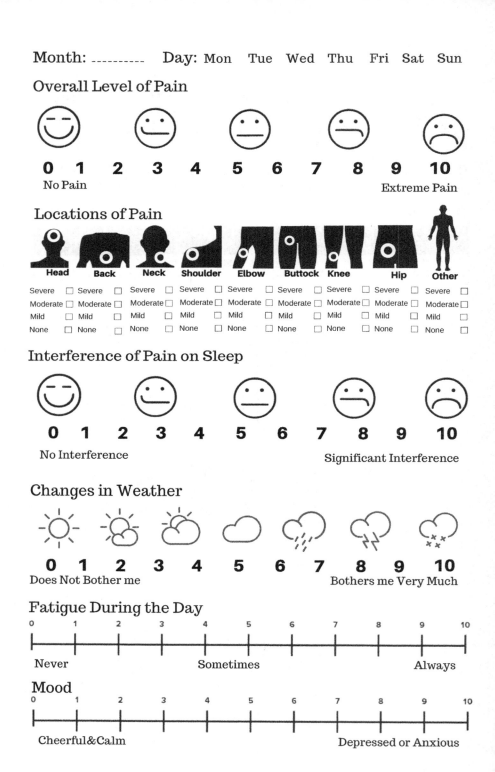

0　1　2　3　4　5　6　7　8　9　10

No Pain

Extreme Pain

Locations of Pain

	Head		Back		Neck		Shoulder		Elbow		Buttock		Knee		Hip		Other
Severe ☐		Severe ☐		Severe ☐		Severe ☐		Severe ☐		Severe ☐		Severe ☐		Severe ☐		Severe ☐
Moderate ☐		Moderate ☐		Moderate ☐		Moderate ☐		Moderate ☐		Moderate ☐		Moderate ☐		Moderate ☐		Moderate ☐
Mild ☐		Mild ☐		Mild ☐		Mild ☐		Mild ☐		Mild ☐		Mild ☐		Mild ☐		Mild ☐
None ☐		None ☐		None ☐		None ☐		None ☐		None ☐		None ☐		None ☐		None ☐

Interference of Pain on Sleep

0　1　2　3　4　5　6　7　8　9　10

No Interference

Significant Interference

Changes in Weather

0　1　2　3　4　5　6　7　8　9　10

Does Not Bother me

Bothers me Very Much

Fatigue During the Day

0　1　2　3　4　5　6　7　8　9　10

Never　　　　　　Sometimes　　　　　　Always

Mood

0　1　2　3　4　5　6　7　8　9　10

Cheerful&Calm

Depressed or Anxious

Exercise

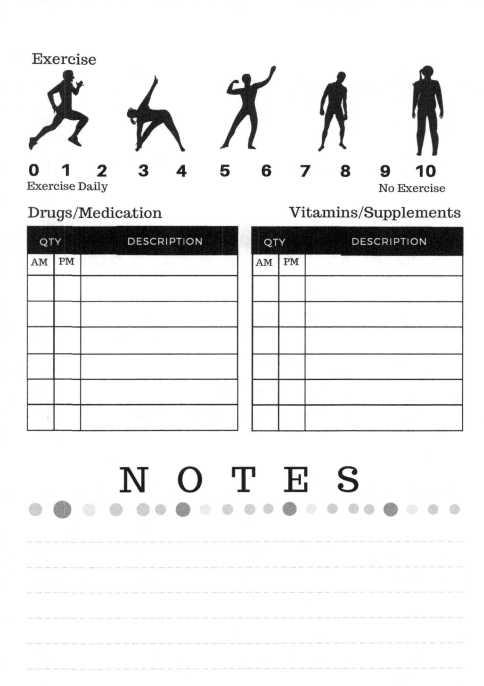

0 1 2   3 4   5   6   7 8   9 10

Exercise Daily   No Exercise

Drugs/Medication

QTY		DESCRIPTION
AM	PM	

Vitamins/Supplements

QTY		DESCRIPTION
AM	PM	

N O T E S

Month: _____ Day: Mon Tue Wed Thu Fri Sat Sun

Overall Level of Pain

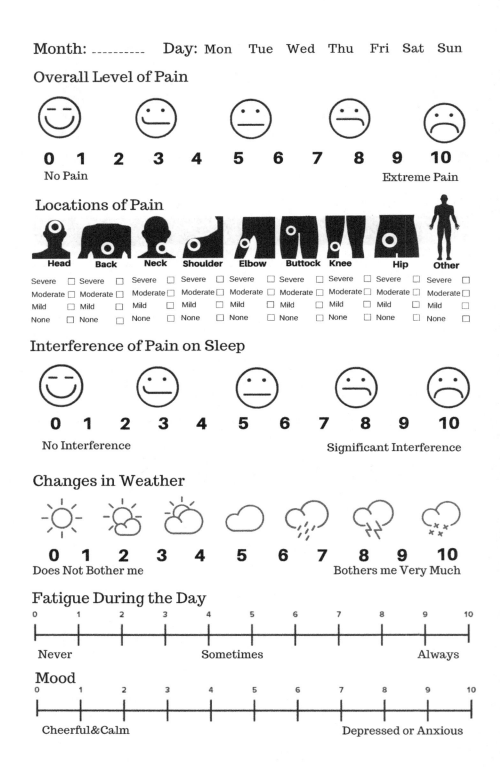

0 1 2 3 4 5 6 7 8 9 10

No Pain   Extreme Pain

Locations of Pain

	Head	Back	Neck	Shoulder	Elbow	Buttock	Knee	Hip	Other
Severe ☐	Severe ☐	Severe ☐	Severe ☐	Severe ☐	Severe ☐	Severe ☐	Severe ☐	Severe ☐	Severe ☐
Moderate ☐	Moderate ☐	Moderate ☐	Moderate ☐	Moderate ☐	Moderate ☐	Moderate ☐	Moderate ☐	Moderate ☐	Moderate ☐
Mild ☐	Mild ☐	Mild ☐	Mild ☐	Mild ☐	Mild ☐	Mild ☐	Mild ☐	Mild ☐	Mild ☐
None ☐	None ☐	None ☐	None ☐	None ☐	None ☐	None ☐	None ☐	None ☐	None ☐

Interference of Pain on Sleep

0 1 2 3 4 5 6 7 8 9 10

No Interference   Significant Interference

Changes in Weather

0 1 2 3 4 5 6 7 8 9 10

Does Not Bother me   Bothers me Very Much

Fatigue During the Day

0   1   2   3   4   5   6   7   8   9   10

Never   Sometimes   Always

Mood

0   1   2   3   4   5   6   7   8   9   10

Cheerful&Calm   Depressed or Anxious

Exercise

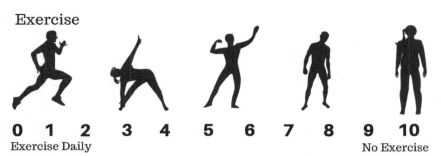

0   1   2   3   4   5   6   7   8   9   10

Exercise Daily   No Exercise

Drugs/Medication

QTY		DESCRIPTION
AM	PM	

Vitamins/Supplements

QTY		DESCRIPTION
AM	PM	

N O T E S

Month: _____ **Day:** Mon Tue Wed Thu Fri Sat Sun

Overall Level of Pain

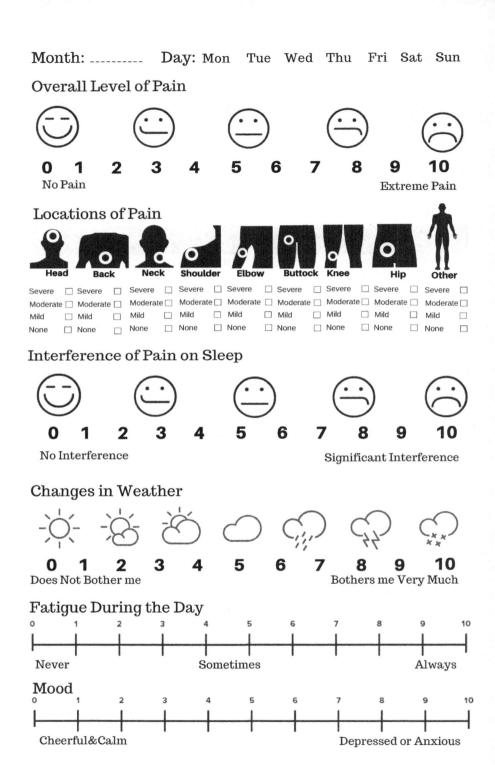

0 1 2 3 4 5 6 7 8 9 10

No Pain   Extreme Pain

Locations of Pain

Head **Back** **Neck** **Shoulder** **Elbow** **Buttock** **Knee** **Hip** **Other**

	Head	Back	Neck	Shoulder	Elbow	Buttock	Knee	Hip	Other
Severe	☐	☐	☐	☐	☐	☐	☐	☐	☐
Moderate	☐	☐	☐	☐	☐	☐	☐	☐	☐
Mild	☐	☐	☐	☐	☐	☐	☐	☐	☐
None	☐	☐	☐	☐	☐	☐	☐	☐	☐

Interference of Pain on Sleep

0 1 2 3 4 5 6 7 8 9 10

No Interference   Significant Interference

Changes in Weather

0 1 2 3 4 5 6 7 8 9 10

Does Not Bother me   Bothers me Very Much

Fatigue During the Day

0   1   2   3   4   5   6   7   8   9   10

Never   Sometimes   Always

Mood

0   1   2   3   4   5   6   7   8   9   10

Cheerful&Calm   Depressed or Anxious

Exercise

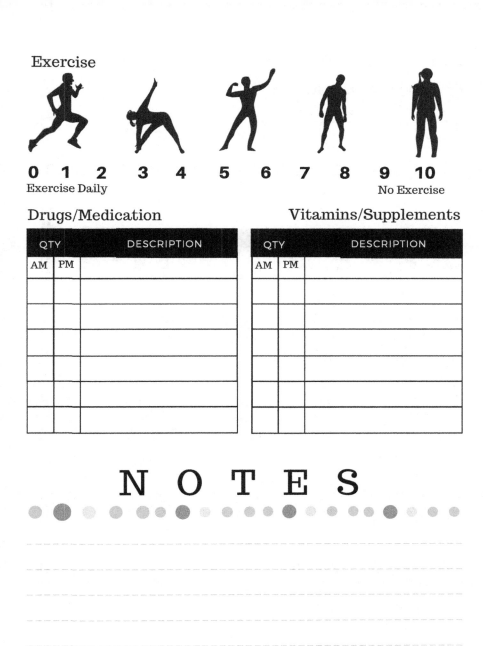

| 0 | 1 | 2 | 3 | 4 | 5 | 6 | 7 | 8 | 9 | 10 |

Exercise Daily · · · · · · · · · · · · · · · · · No Exercise

Drugs/Medication

QTY		DESCRIPTION
AM	PM	

Vitamins/Supplements

QTY		DESCRIPTION
AM	PM	

N O T E S

Month: ---------- **Day:** Mon Tue Wed Thu Fri Sat Sun

Overall Level of Pain

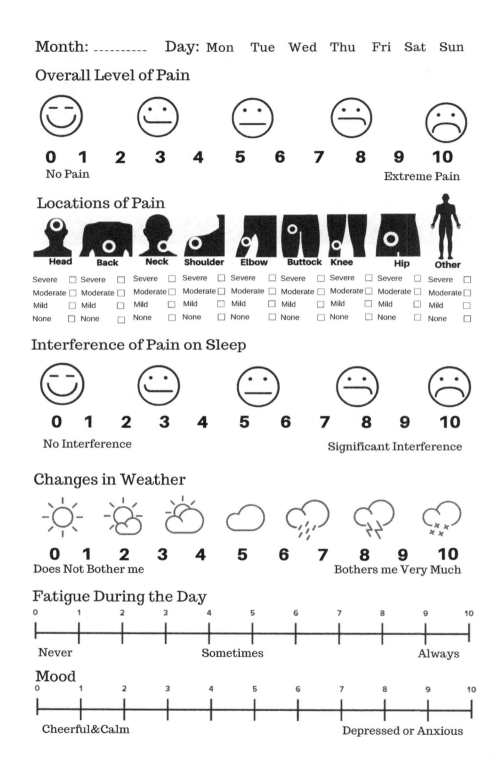

0 1 2 3 4 5 6 7 8 9 10

No Pain   Extreme Pain

Locations of Pain

	Head	Back	Neck	Shoulder	Elbow	Buttock	Knee	Hip	Other
Severe	☐	☐	☐	☐	☐	☐	☐	☐	☐
Moderate	☐	☐	☐	☐	☐	☐	☐	☐	☐
Mild	☐	☐	☐	☐	☐	☐	☐	☐	☐
None	☐	☐	☐	☐	☐	☐	☐	☐	☐

Interference of Pain on Sleep

0 1 2 3 4 5 6 7 8 9 10

No Interference   Significant Interference

Changes in Weather

0 1 2 3 4 5 6 7 8 9 10

Does Not Bother me   Bothers me Very Much

Fatigue During the Day

0 1 2 3 4 5 6 7 8 9 10

Never   Sometimes   Always

Mood

0 1 2 3 4 5 6 7 8 9 10

Cheerful&Calm   Depressed or Anxious

Exercise

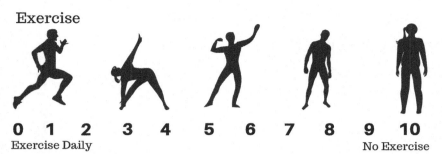

0 1 2   3   4   5   6   7   8   9 10

Exercise Daily   No Exercise

Drugs/Medication

QTY		DESCRIPTION
AM	PM	

Vitamins/Supplements

QTY		DESCRIPTION
AM	PM	

N O T E S

Month: _____ **Day:** Mon Tue Wed Thu Fri Sat Sun

Overall Level of Pain

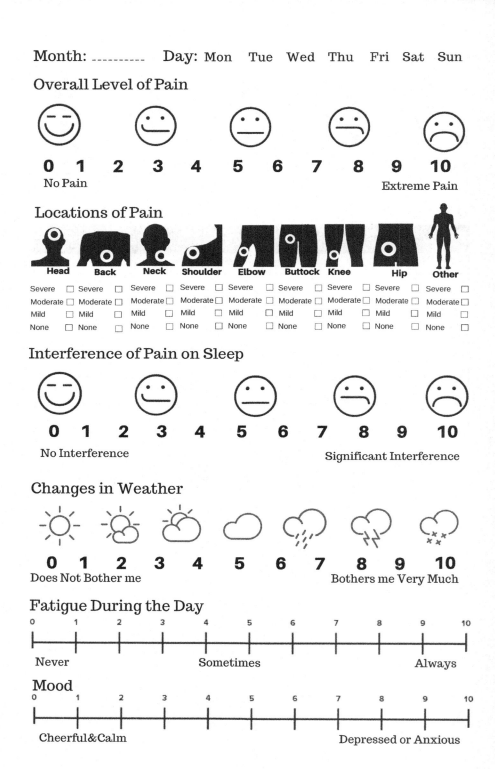

0   1   2   3   4   5   6   7   8   9   10

No Pain   Extreme Pain

Locations of Pain

Head   Back   Neck   Shoulder   Elbow   Buttock   Knee   Hip   Other

Severe ☐	Severe ☐	Severe ☐	Severe ☐	Severe ☐	Severe ☐	Severe ☐	Severe ☐	Severe ☐
Moderate ☐	Moderate ☐	Moderate ☐	Moderate ☐	Moderate ☐	Moderate ☐	Moderate ☐	Moderate ☐	Moderate ☐
Mild ☐	Mild ☐	Mild ☐	Mild ☐	Mild ☐	Mild ☐	Mild ☐	Mild ☐	Mild ☐
None ☐	None ☐	None ☐	None ☐	None ☐	None ☐	None ☐	None ☐	None ☐

Interference of Pain on Sleep

0   1   2   3   4   5   6   7   8   9   10

No Interference   Significant Interference

Changes in Weather

0   1   2   3   4   5   6   7   8   9   10

Does Not Bother me   Bothers me Very Much

Fatigue During the Day

0   1   2   3   4   5   6   7   8   9   10

Never   Sometimes   Always

Mood

0   1   2   3   4   5   6   7   8   9   10

Cheerful&Calm   Depressed or Anxious

Exercise

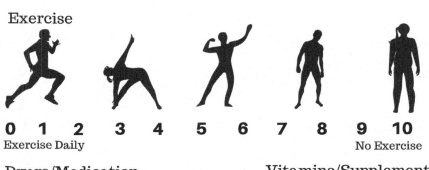

0   1   2   3   4   5   6   7   8   9   10

Exercise Daily   No Exercise

Drugs/Medication

QTY		DESCRIPTION
AM	PM	

Vitamins/Supplements

QTY		DESCRIPTION
AM	PM	

N O T E S

Month: _____ **Day:** Mon   Tue   Wed   Thu   Fri   Sat   Sun

Overall Level of Pain

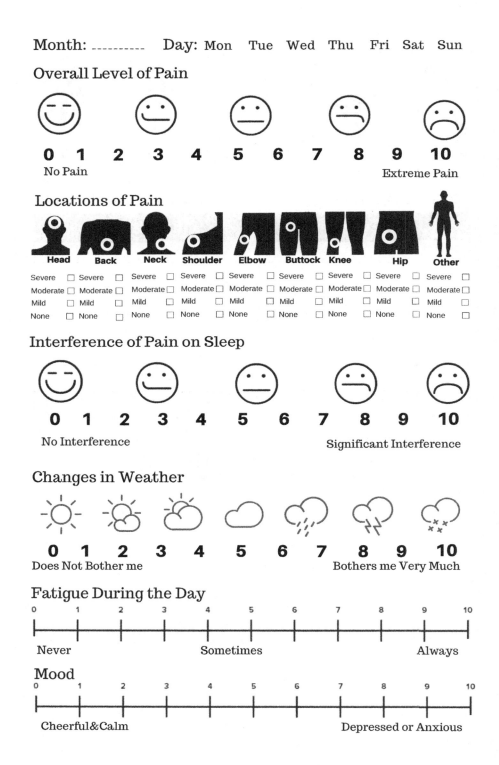

0   1   2   3   4   5   6   7   8   9   10

No Pain   Extreme Pain

Locations of Pain

	Head	Back	Neck	Shoulder	Elbow	Buttock	Knee	Hip	Other
Severe	☐	☐	☐	☐	☐	☐	☐	☐	☐
Moderate	☐	☐	☐	☐	☐	☐	☐	☐	☐
Mild	☐	☐	☐	☐	☐	☐	☐	☐	☐
None	☐	☐	☐	☐	☐	☐	☐	☐	☐

Interference of Pain on Sleep

0   1   2   3   4   5   6   7   8   9   10

No Interference   Significant Interference

Changes in Weather

0   1   2   3   4   5   6   7   8   9   10

Does Not Bother me   Bothers me Very Much

Fatigue During the Day

0   1   2   3   4   5   6   7   8   9   10

Never   Sometimes   Always

Mood

0   1   2   3   4   5   6   7   8   9   10

Cheerful&Calm   Depressed or Anxious

Exercise

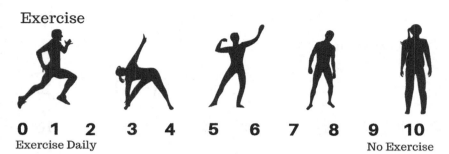

0   1   2   3   4   5   6   7   8   9   10

Exercise Daily   No Exercise

Drugs/Medication

QTY		DESCRIPTION
AM	PM	

Vitamins/Supplements

QTY		DESCRIPTION
AM	PM	

N O T E S

Month: ---------- **Day:** Mon Tue Wed Thu Fri Sat Sun

Overall Level of Pain

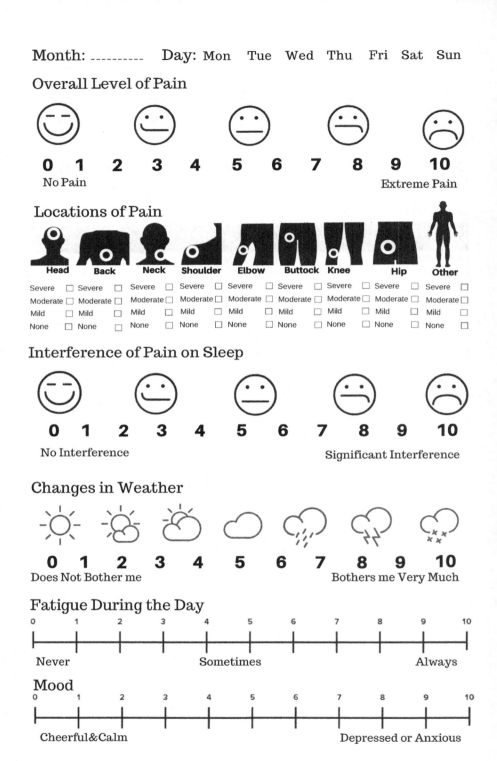

0 1 2 3 4 5 6 7 8 9 10

No Pain   Extreme Pain

Locations of Pain

Head Back Neck Shoulder Elbow Buttock Knee Hip Other

Severe ☐	Severe ☐	Severe ☐	Severe ☐	Severe ☐	Severe ☐	Severe ☐	Severe ☐	Severe ☐
Moderate ☐	Moderate ☐	Moderate ☐	Moderate ☐	Moderate ☐	Moderate ☐	Moderate ☐	Moderate ☐	Moderate ☐
Mild ☐	Mild ☐	Mild ☐	Mild ☐	Mild ☐	Mild ☐	Mild ☐	Mild ☐	Mild ☐
None ☐	None ☐	None ☐	None ☐	None ☐	None ☐	None ☐	None ☐	None ☐

Interference of Pain on Sleep

0 1 2 3 4 5 6 7 8 9 10

No Interference   Significant Interference

Changes in Weather

0 1 2 3 4 5 6 7 8 9 10

Does Not Bother me   Bothers me Very Much

Fatigue During the Day

0   1   2   3   4   5   6   7   8   9   10

Never   Sometimes   Always

Mood

0   1   2   3   4   5   6   7   8   9   10

Cheerful&Calm   Depressed or Anxious

Exercise

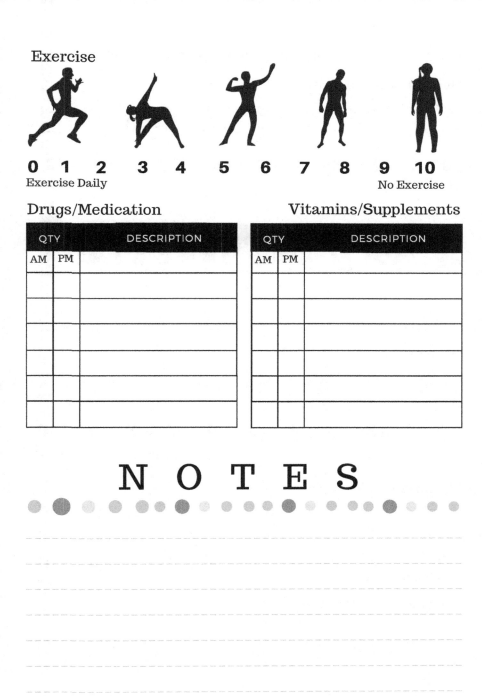

0 1 2 3 4 5 6 7 8 9 10

Exercise Daily   No Exercise

Drugs/Medication

QTY		DESCRIPTION
AM	PM	

Vitamins/Supplements

QTY		DESCRIPTION
AM	PM	

N O T E S

Month: ---------- Day: Mon Tue Wed Thu Fri Sat Sun

Overall Level of Pain

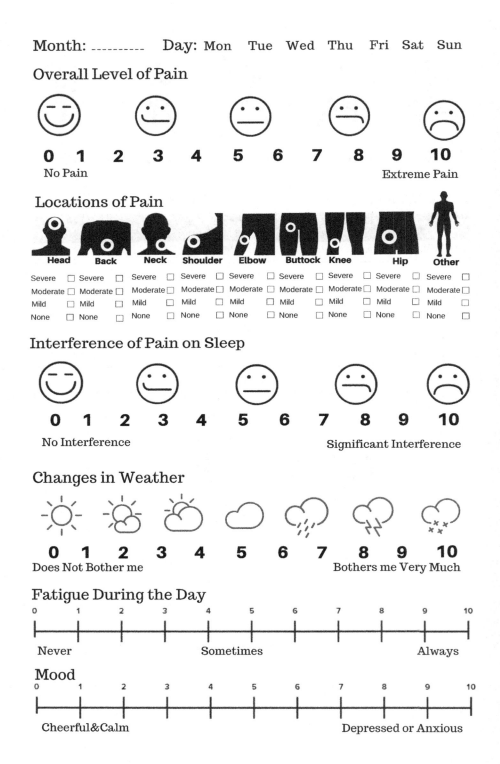

| 0 | 1 | 2 | 3 | 4 | 5 | 6 | 7 | 8 | 9 | 10 |

No Pain   Extreme Pain

Locations of Pain

Head	Back	Neck	Shoulder	Elbow	Buttock	Knee	Hip	Other
Severe ☐	Severe ☐	Severe ☐	Severe ☐	Severe ☐	Severe ☐	Severe ☐	Severe ☐	Severe ☐
Moderate ☐	Moderate ☐	Moderate ☐	Moderate ☐	Moderate ☐	Moderate ☐	Moderate ☐	Moderate ☐	Moderate ☐
Mild ☐	Mild ☐	Mild ☐	Mild ☐	Mild ☐	Mild ☐	Mild ☐	Mild ☐	Mild ☐
None ☐	None ☐	None ☐	None ☐	None ☐	None ☐	None ☐	None ☐	None ☐

Interference of Pain on Sleep

| 0 | 1 | 2 | 3 | 4 | 5 | 6 | 7 | 8 | 9 | 10 |

No Interference   Significant Interference

Changes in Weather

| 0 | 1 | 2 | 3 | 4 | 5 | 6 | 7 | 8 | 9 | 10 |

Does Not Bother me   Bothers me Very Much

Fatigue During the Day

0   1   2   3   4   5   6   7   8   9   10

Never   Sometimes   Always

Mood

0   1   2   3   4   5   6   7   8   9   10

Cheerful&Calm   Depressed or Anxious

Exercise

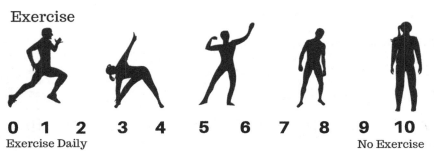

| 0 | 1 | 2 | 3 | 4 | 5 | 6 | 7 | 8 | 9 | 10 |

Exercise Daily   No Exercise

Drugs/Medication

QTY		DESCRIPTION
AM	PM	

Vitamins/Supplements

QTY		DESCRIPTION
AM	PM	

N O T E S

Month: _____ **Day:** Mon Tue Wed Thu Fri Sat Sun

Overall Level of Pain

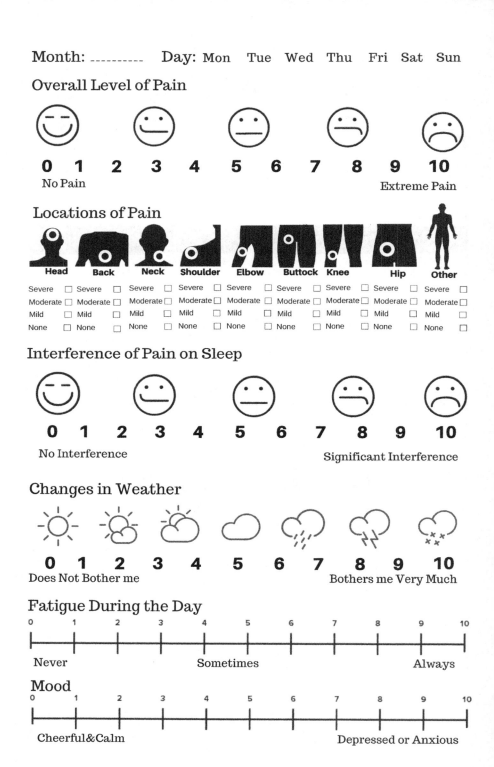

0   1   2   3   4   5   6   7   8   9   10

No Pain   Extreme Pain

Locations of Pain

	Head	Back	Neck	Shoulder	Elbow	Buttock	Knee	Hip	Other
Severe	☐	☐	☐	☐	☐	☐	☐	☐	☐
Moderate	☐	☐	☐	☐	☐	☐	☐	☐	☐
Mild	☐	☐	☐	☐	☐	☐	☐	☐	☐
None	☐	☐	☐	☐	☐	☐	☐	☐	☐

Interference of Pain on Sleep

0   1   2   3   4   5   6   7   8   9   10

No Interference   Significant Interference

Changes in Weather

0   1   2   3   4   5   6   7   8   9   10

Does Not Bother me   Bothers me Very Much

Fatigue During the Day

0   1   2   3   4   5   6   7   8   9   10

Never   Sometimes   Always

Mood

0   1   2   3   4   5   6   7   8   9   10

Cheerful&Calm   Depressed or Anxious

Exercise

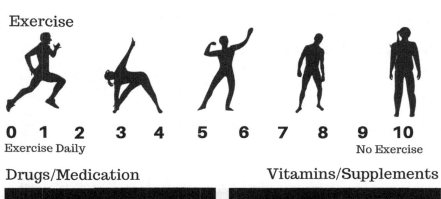

| 0 | 1 | 2 | 3 | 4 | 5 | 6 | 7 | 8 | 9 | 10 |

Exercise Daily   No Exercise

Drugs/Medication

QTY		DESCRIPTION
AM	PM	

Vitamins/Supplements

QTY		DESCRIPTION
AM	PM	

N O T E S

Month: _____ Day: Mon Tue Wed Thu Fri Sat Sun

Overall Level of Pain

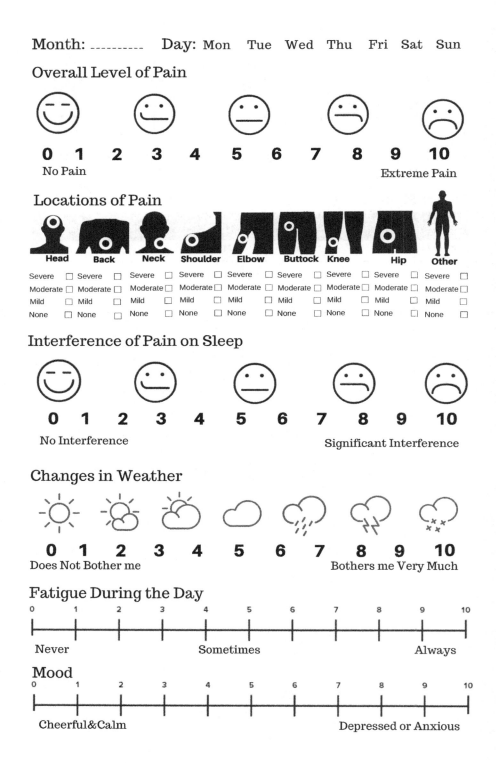

0 1   2   3   4   5   6   7   8   9   10

No Pain   Extreme Pain

Locations of Pain

Head   Back   Neck   Shoulder   Elbow   Buttock   Knee   Hip   Other

	Head	Back	Neck	Shoulder	Elbow	Buttock	Knee	Hip	Other
Severe	☐	☐	☐	☐	☐	☐	☐	☐	☐
Moderate	☐	☐	☐	☐	☐	☐	☐	☐	☐
Mild	☐	☐	☐	☐	☐	☐	☐	☐	☐
None	☐	☐	☐	☐	☐	☐	☐	☐	☐

Interference of Pain on Sleep

0 1   2   3   4   5   6   7   8   9   10

No Interference   Significant Interference

Changes in Weather

0 1   2   3   4   5   6   7   8   9   10

Does Not Bother me   Bothers me Very Much

Fatigue During the Day

0   1   2   3   4   5   6   7   8   9   10

Never   Sometimes   Always

Mood

0   1   2   3   4   5   6   7   8   9   10

Cheerful&Calm   Depressed or Anxious

Exercise

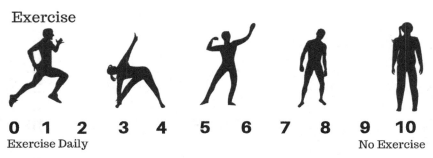

0 1 2   3   4   5   6   7   8   9 10

Exercise Daily   No Exercise

Drugs/Medication

QTY		DESCRIPTION
AM	PM	

Vitamins/Supplements

QTY		DESCRIPTION
AM	PM	

N O T E S

Month: ---------- Day: Mon Tue Wed Thu Fri Sat Sun

Overall Level of Pain

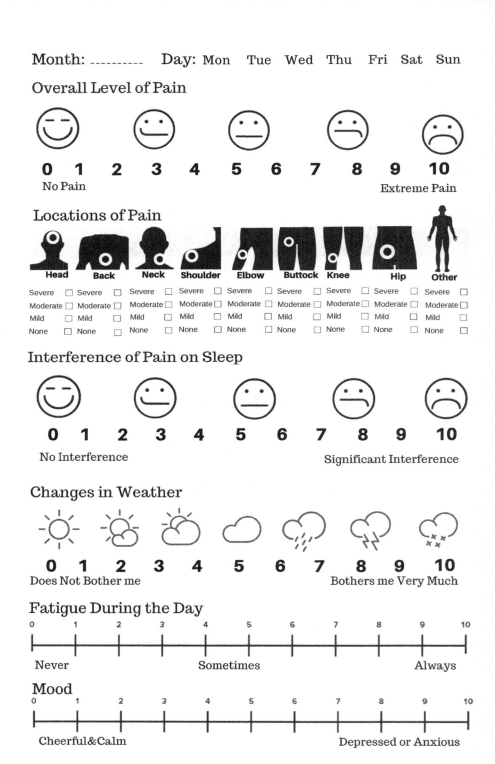

0 1 2 3 4 5 6 7 8 9 10

No Pain

Extreme Pain

Locations of Pain

	Head	Back	Neck	Shoulder	Elbow	Buttock	Knee	Hip	Other
Severe	☐	☐	☐	☐	☐	☐	☐	☐	☐
Moderate	☐	☐	☐	☐	☐	☐	☐	☐	☐
Mild	☐	☐	☐	☐	☐	☐	☐	☐	☐
None	☐	☐	☐	☐	☐	☐	☐	☐	☐

Interference of Pain on Sleep

0 1 2 3 4 5 6 7 8 9 10

No Interference

Significant Interference

Changes in Weather

0 1 2 3 4 5 6 7 8 9 10

Does Not Bother me

Bothers me Very Much

Fatigue During the Day

0 1 2 3 4 5 6 7 8 9 10

Never   Sometimes   Always

Mood

0 1 2 3 4 5 6 7 8 9 10

Cheerful&Calm   Depressed or Anxious

Exercise

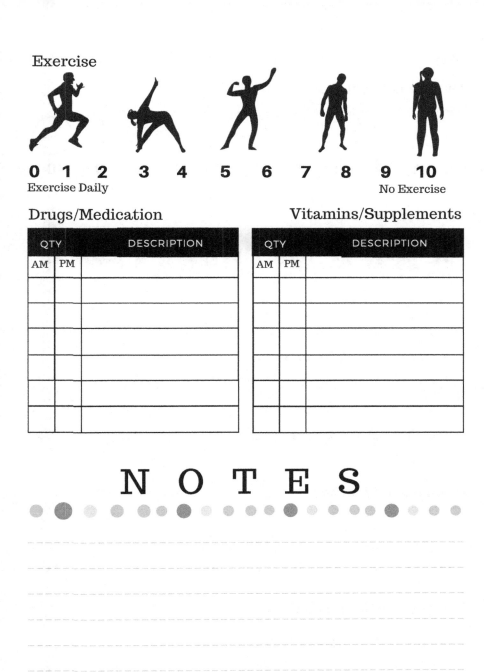

0   1   2   3   4   5   6   7   8   9   10

Exercise Daily   No Exercise

Drugs/Medication

QTY		DESCRIPTION
AM	PM	

Vitamins/Supplements

QTY		DESCRIPTION
AM	PM	

N O T E S

Month: ---------- **Day:** Mon Tue Wed Thu Fri Sat Sun

Overall Level of Pain

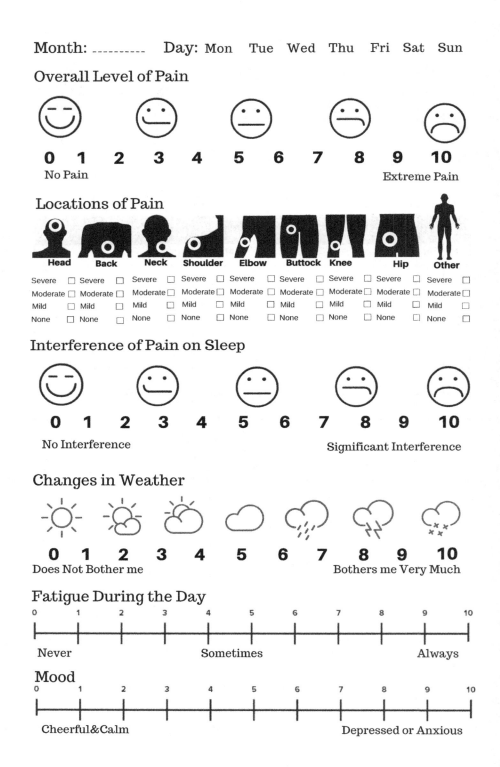

0 1 2 3 4 5 6 7 8 9 10

No Pain   Extreme Pain

Locations of Pain

	Head	Back	Neck	Shoulder	Elbow	Buttock	Knee	Hip	Other
Severe	☐	☐	☐	☐	☐	☐	☐	☐	☐
Moderate	☐	☐	☐	☐	☐	☐	☐	☐	☐
Mild	☐	☐	☐	☐	☐	☐	☐	☐	☐
None	☐	☐	☐	☐	☐	☐	☐	☐	☐

Interference of Pain on Sleep

0 1 2 3 4 5 6 7 8 9 10

No Interference   Significant Interference

Changes in Weather

0 1 2 3 4 5 6 7 8 9 10

Does Not Bother me   Bothers me Very Much

Fatigue During the Day

0   1   2   3   4   5   6   7   8   9   10

Never   Sometimes   Always

Mood

0   1   2   3   4   5   6   7   8   9   10

Cheerful&Calm   Depressed or Anxious

Exercise

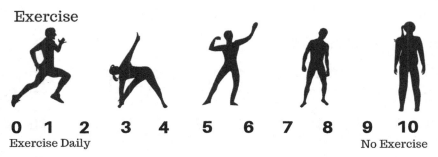

0 1 2   3   4   5   6   7   8   9   10

Exercise Daily   No Exercise

Drugs/Medication

QTY		DESCRIPTION
AM	PM	

Vitamins/Supplements

QTY		DESCRIPTION
AM	PM	

N O T E S

Month: ---------- **Day:** Mon   Tue   Wed   Thu   Fri   Sat   Sun

Overall Level of Pain

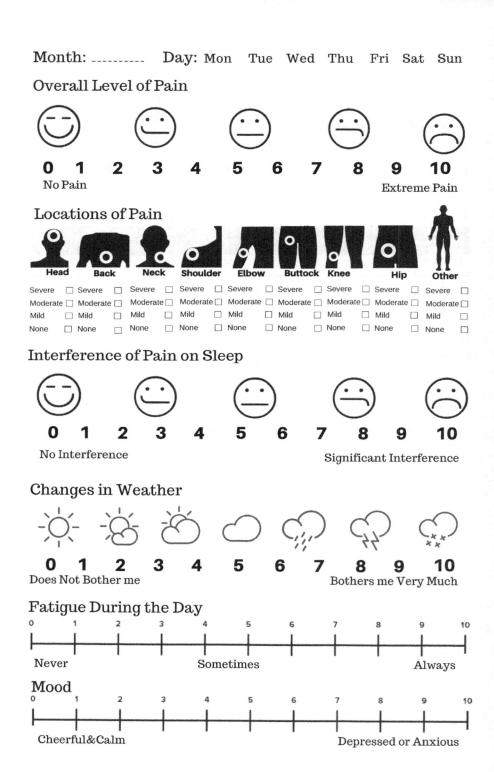

0   1   2   3   4   5   6   7   8   9   10

No Pain   Extreme Pain

Locations of Pain

	Head	Back	Neck	Shoulder	Elbow	Buttock	Knee	Hip	Other
Severe	☐	☐	☐	☐	☐	☐	☐	☐	☐
Moderate	☐	☐	☐	☐	☐	☐	☐	☐	☐
Mild	☐	☐	☐	☐	☐	☐	☐	☐	☐
None	☐	☐	☐	☐	☐	☐	☐	☐	☐

Interference of Pain on Sleep

0   1   2   3   4   5   6   7   8   9   10

No Interference   Significant Interference

Changes in Weather

0   1   2   3   4   5   6   7   8   9   10

Does Not Bother me   Bothers me Very Much

Fatigue During the Day

0   1   2   3   4   5   6   7   8   9   10

Never   Sometimes   Always

Mood

0   1   2   3   4   5   6   7   8   9   10

Cheerful&Calm   Depressed or Anxious

Exercise

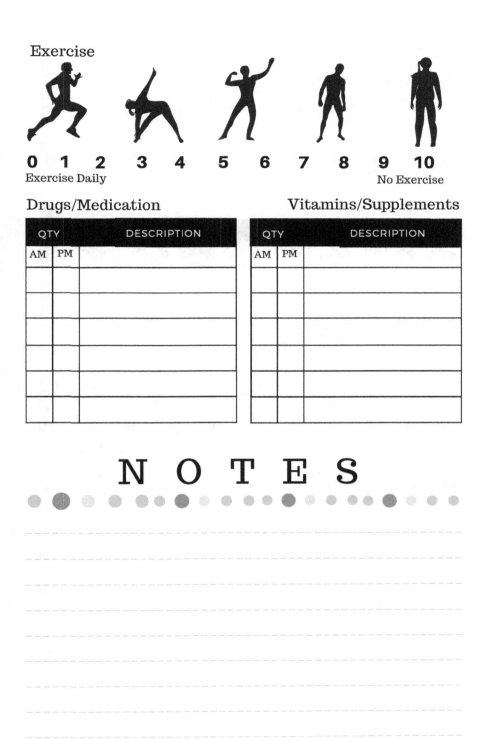

0 1 2 3 4 5 6 7 8 9 10

Exercise Daily   No Exercise

Drugs/Medication

QTY		DESCRIPTION
AM	PM	

Vitamins/Supplements

QTY		DESCRIPTION
AM	PM	

N O T E S

Month: ---------- **Day:** Mon   Tue   Wed   Thu   Fri   Sat   Sun

Overall Level of Pain

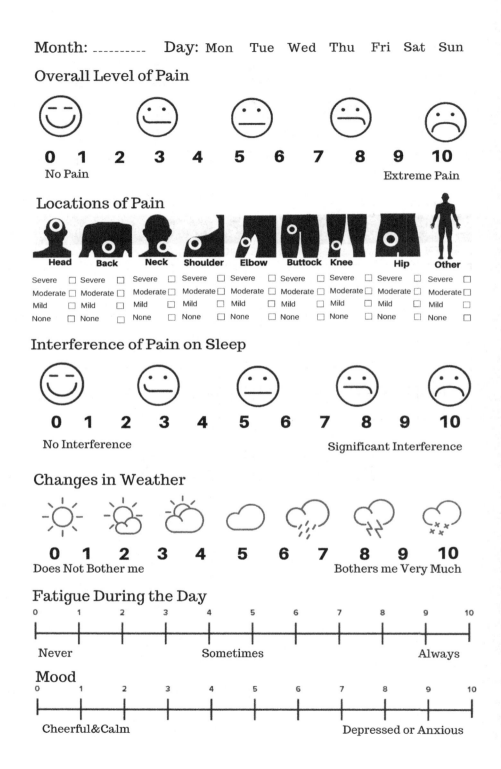

0   1   2   3   4   5   6   7   8   9   10

No Pain   Extreme Pain

Locations of Pain

Head	Back	Neck	Shoulder	Elbow	Buttock	Knee	Hip	Other
Severe ☐	Severe ☐	Severe ☐	Severe ☐	Severe ☐	Severe ☐	Severe ☐	Severe ☐	Severe ☐
Moderate ☐	Moderate ☐	Moderate ☐	Moderate ☐	Moderate ☐	Moderate ☐	Moderate ☐	Moderate ☐	Moderate ☐
Mild ☐	Mild ☐	Mild ☐	Mild ☐	Mild ☐	Mild ☐	Mild ☐	Mild ☐	Mild ☐
None ☐	None ☐	None ☐	None ☐	None ☐	None ☐	None ☐	None ☐	None ☐

Interference of Pain on Sleep

0   1   2   3   4   5   6   7   8   9   10

No Interference   Significant Interference

Changes in Weather

0   1   2   3   4   5   6   7   8   9   10

Does Not Bother me   Bothers me Very Much

Fatigue During the Day

0   1   2   3   4   5   6   7   8   9   10

Never   Sometimes   Always

Mood

0   1   2   3   4   5   6   7   8   9   10

Cheerful&Calm   Depressed or Anxious

Exercise

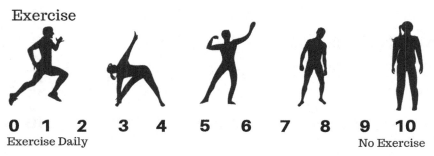

0 1 2   3   4   5   6   7   8   9 10

Exercise Daily   No Exercise

Drugs/Medication

QTY		DESCRIPTION
AM	PM	

Vitamins/Supplements

QTY		DESCRIPTION
AM	PM	

N O T E S

Month: .... **Day:** Mon Tue Wed Thu Fri Sat Sun

Overall Level of Pain

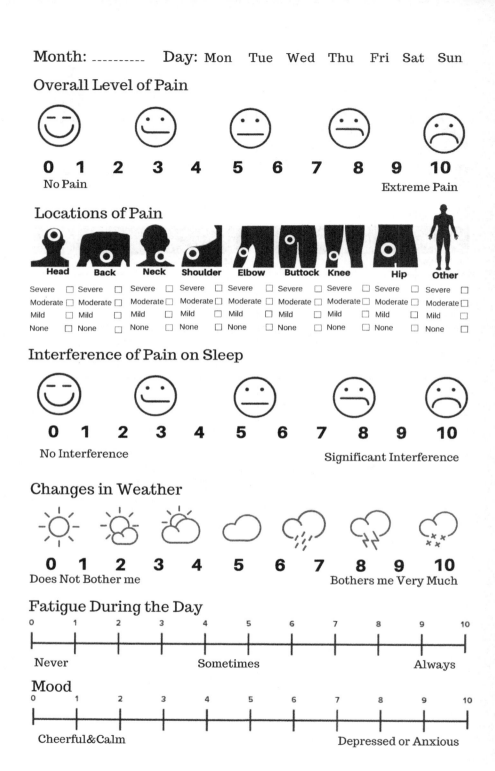

0   1   2   3   4   5   6   7   8   9   10

No Pain   Extreme Pain

Locations of Pain

Head	Back	Neck	Shoulder	Elbow	Buttock	Knee	Hip	Other
Severe ☐	Severe ☐	Severe ☐	Severe ☐	Severe ☐	Severe ☐	Severe ☐	Severe ☐	Severe ☐
Moderate ☐	Moderate ☐	Moderate ☐	Moderate ☐	Moderate ☐	Moderate ☐	Moderate ☐	Moderate ☐	Moderate ☐
Mild ☐	Mild ☐	Mild ☐	Mild ☐	Mild ☐	Mild ☐	Mild ☐	Mild ☐	Mild ☐
None ☐	None ☐	None ☐	None ☐	None ☐	None ☐	None ☐	None ☐	None ☐

Interference of Pain on Sleep

0   1   2   3   4   5   6   7   8   9   10

No Interference   Significant Interference

Changes in Weather

0   1   2   3   4   5   6   7   8   9   10

Does Not Bother me   Bothers me Very Much

Fatigue During the Day

0   1   2   3   4   5   6   7   8   9   10

Never   Sometimes   Always

Mood

0   1   2   3   4   5   6   7   8   9   10

Cheerful&Calm   Depressed or Anxious

Exercise

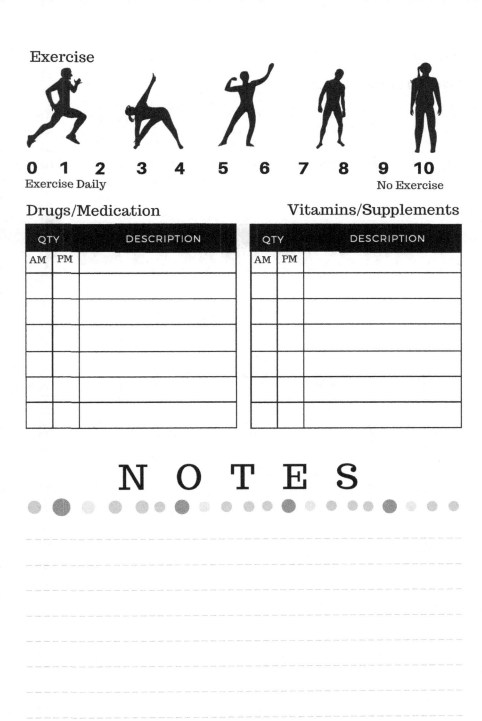

0   1   2   3   4   5   6   7   8   9   10

Exercise Daily   No Exercise

Drugs/Medication

QTY		DESCRIPTION
AM	PM	

Vitamins/Supplements

QTY		DESCRIPTION
AM	PM	

N O T E S

Month: ---------- **Day:** Mon Tue Wed Thu Fri Sat Sun

Overall Level of Pain

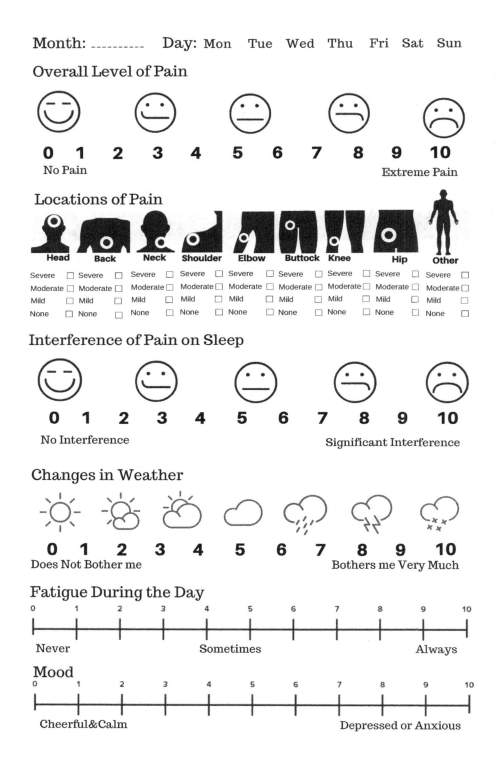

0 1 2 3 4 5 6 7 8 9 10

No Pain   Extreme Pain

Locations of Pain

Head   Back   Neck   Shoulder   Elbow   Buttock   Knee   Hip   Other

	Head	Back	Neck	Shoulder	Elbow	Buttock	Knee	Hip	Other
Severe	☐	☐	☐	☐	☐	☐	☐	☐	☐
Moderate	☐	☐	☐	☐	☐	☐	☐	☐	☐
Mild	☐	☐	☐	☐	☐	☐	☐	☐	☐
None	☐	☐	☐	☐	☐	☐	☐	☐	☐

Interference of Pain on Sleep

0 1 2 3 4 5 6 7 8 9 10

No Interference   Significant Interference

Changes in Weather

0 1 2 3 4 5 6 7 8 9 10

Does Not Bother me   Bothers me Very Much

Fatigue During the Day

0   1   2   3   4   5   6   7   8   9   10

Never   Sometimes   Always

Mood

0   1   2   3   4   5   6   7   8   9   10

Cheerful&Calm   Depressed or Anxious

Exercise

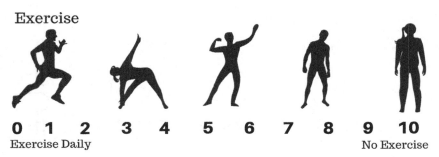

0 1 2   3   4   5   6   7   8   9   10

Exercise Daily   No Exercise

Drugs/Medication

QTY		DESCRIPTION
AM	PM	

Vitamins/Supplements

QTY		DESCRIPTION
AM	PM	

N O T E S

Month: _____ Day: Mon Tue Wed Thu Fri Sat Sun

Overall Level of Pain

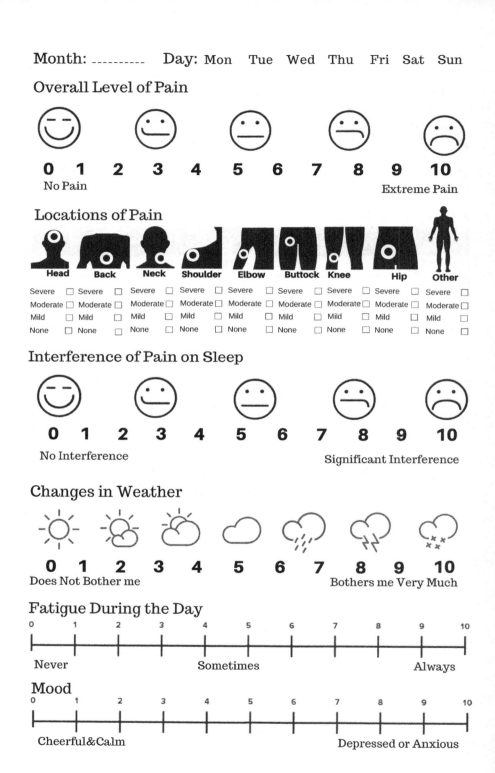

0 1 2 3 4 5 6 7 8 9 10

No Pain

Extreme Pain

Locations of Pain

Head	Back	Neck	Shoulder	Elbow	Buttock	Knee	Hip	Other
Severe ☐	Severe ☐	Severe ☐	Severe ☐	Severe ☐	Severe ☐	Severe ☐	Severe ☐	Severe ☐
Moderate ☐	Moderate ☐	Moderate ☐	Moderate ☐	Moderate ☐	Moderate ☐	Moderate ☐	Moderate ☐	Moderate ☐
Mild ☐	Mild ☐	Mild ☐	Mild ☐	Mild ☐	Mild ☐	Mild ☐	Mild ☐	Mild ☐
None ☐	None ☐	None ☐	None ☐	None ☐	None ☐	None ☐	None ☐	None ☐

Interference of Pain on Sleep

0 1 2 3 4 5 6 7 8 9 10

No Interference

Significant Interference

Changes in Weather

0 1 2 3 4 5 6 7 8 9 10

Does Not Bother me

Bothers me Very Much

Fatigue During the Day

0 1 2 3 4 5 6 7 8 9 10

Never

Sometimes

Always

Mood

0 1 2 3 4 5 6 7 8 9 10

Cheerful&Calm

Depressed or Anxious

Exercise

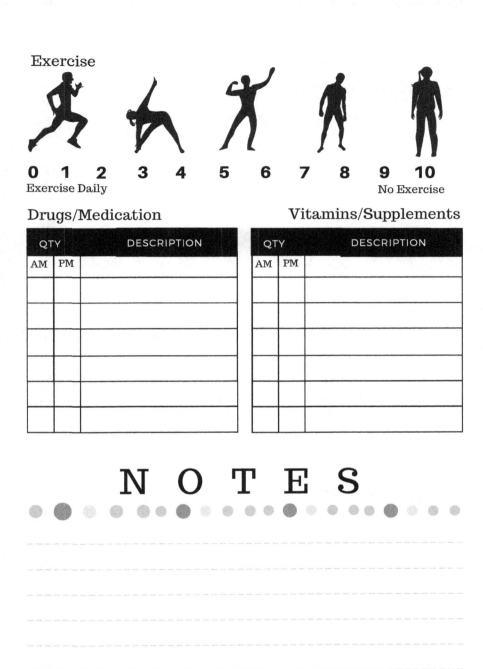

0   1   2   3   4   5   6   7   8   9   10

Exercise Daily   No Exercise

Drugs/Medication

QTY		DESCRIPTION
AM	PM	

Vitamins/Supplements

QTY		DESCRIPTION
AM	PM	

N O T E S

Month: ---------- Day: Mon Tue Wed Thu Fri Sat Sun

Overall Level of Pain

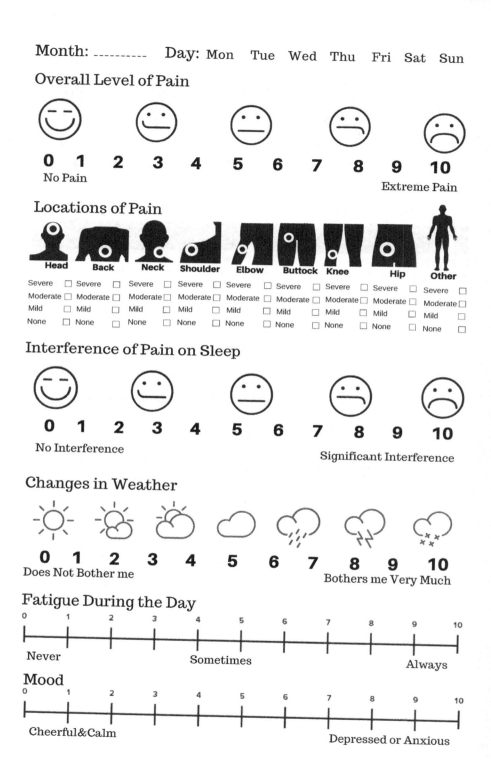

0 1 2 3 4 5 6 7 8 9 10

No Pain

Extreme Pain

Locations of Pain

Head **Back** **Neck** **Shoulder** **Elbow** **Buttock** **Knee** **Hip** **Other**

Head	Back	Neck	Shoulder	Elbow	Buttock	Knee	Hip	Other
Severe ☐	Severe ☐	Severe ☐	Severe ☐	Severe ☐	Severe ☐	Severe ☐	Severe ☐	Severe ☐
Moderate ☐	Moderate ☐	Moderate☐	Moderate☐	Moderate ☐	Moderate ☐	Moderate☐	Moderate ☐	Moderate☐
Mild ☐	Mild ☐	Mild ☐	Mild ☐	Mild ☐	Mild ☐	Mild ☐	Mild ☐	Mild ☐
None ☐	None ☐	None ☐	None ☐	None ☐	None ☐	None ☐	None ☐	None ☐

Interference of Pain on Sleep

0 1 2 3 4 5 6 7 8 9 10

No Interference

Significant Interference

Changes in Weather

0 1 2 3 4 5 6 7 8 9 10

Does Not Bother me

Bothers me Very Much

Fatigue During the Day

0   1   2   3   4   5   6   7   8   9   10

Never   Sometimes   Always

Mood

0   1   2   3   4   5   6   7   8   9   10

Cheerful&Calm   Depressed or Anxious

Exercise

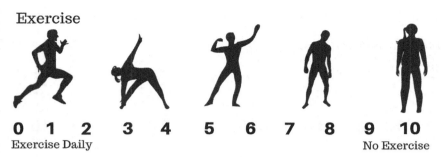

0 1 2 3 4 5 6 7 8 9 10

Exercise Daily   No Exercise

Drugs/Medication

QTY		DESCRIPTION
AM	PM	

Vitamins/Supplements

QTY		DESCRIPTION
AM	PM	

N O T E S

Month: ---------- **Day:** Mon Tue Wed Thu Fri Sat Sun

Overall Level of Pain

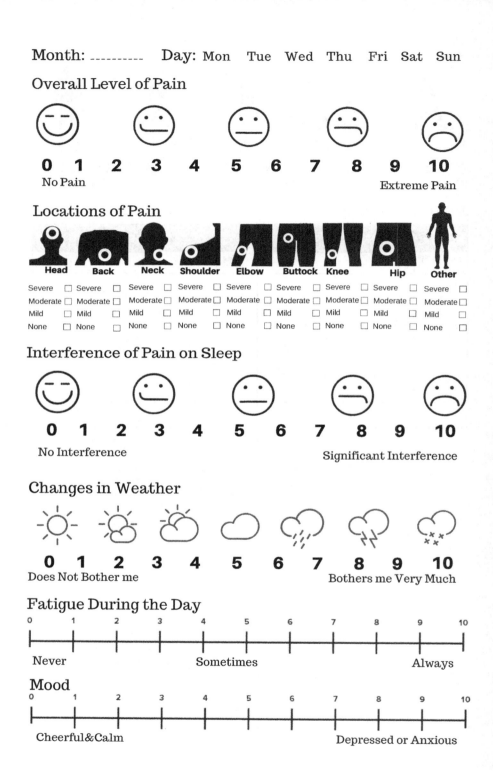

0 1 2 3 4 5 6 7 8 9 10

No Pain   Extreme Pain

Locations of Pain

Head	Back	Neck	Shoulder	Elbow	Buttock	Knee	Hip	Other
Severe ☐	Severe ☐	Severe ☐	Severe ☐	Severe ☐	Severe ☐	Severe ☐	Severe ☐	Severe ☐
Moderate ☐	Moderate ☐	Moderate ☐	Moderate ☐	Moderate ☐	Moderate ☐	Moderate ☐	Moderate ☐	Moderate ☐
Mild ☐	Mild ☐	Mild ☐	Mild ☐	Mild ☐	Mild ☐	Mild ☐	Mild ☐	Mild ☐
None ☐	None ☐	None ☐	None ☐	None ☐	None ☐	None ☐	None ☐	None ☐

Interference of Pain on Sleep

0 1 2 3 4 5 6 7 8 9 10

No Interference   Significant Interference

Changes in Weather

0 1 2 3 4 5 6 7 8 9 10

Does Not Bother me   Bothers me Very Much

Fatigue During the Day

0   1   2   3   4   5   6   7   8   9   10

Never   Sometimes   Always

Mood

0   1   2   3   4   5   6   7   8   9   10

Cheerful&Calm   Depressed or Anxious

Exercise

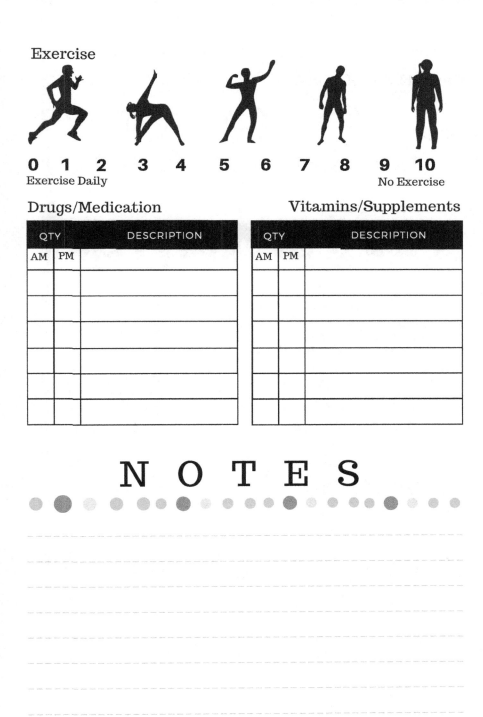

0 1 2 3 4 5 6 7 8 9 10

Exercise Daily   No Exercise

Drugs/Medication

QTY		DESCRIPTION
AM	PM	

Vitamins/Supplements

QTY		DESCRIPTION
AM	PM	

N O T E S

Month: ---------- **Day:** Mon   Tue   Wed   Thu   Fri   Sat   Sun

Overall Level of Pain

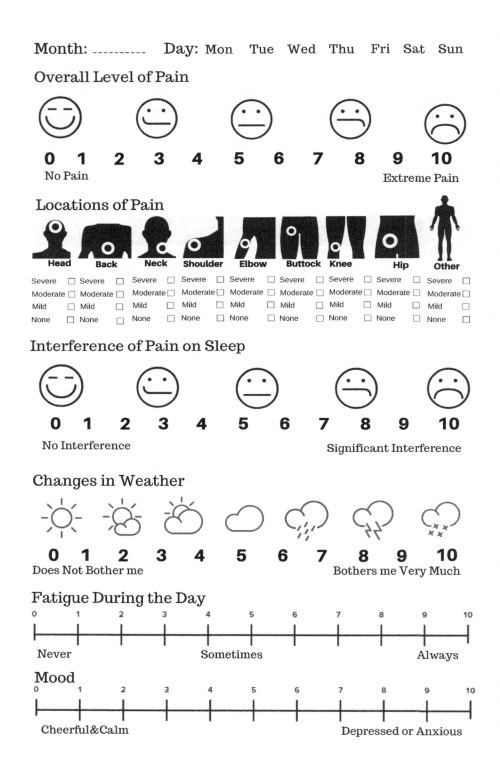

0 1 2 3 4 5 6 7 8 9 10

No Pain   Extreme Pain

Locations of Pain

	Head	Back	Neck	Shoulder	Elbow	Buttock	Knee	Hip	Other
Severe	☐	☐	☐	☐	☐	☐	☐	☐	☐
Moderate	☐	☐	☐	☐	☐	☐	☐	☐	☐
Mild	☐	☐	☐	☐	☐	☐	☐	☐	☐
None	☐	☐	☐	☐	☐	☐	☐	☐	☐

Interference of Pain on Sleep

0 1 2 3 4 5 6 7 8 9 10

No Interference   Significant Interference

Changes in Weather

0 1 2 3 4 5 6 7 8 9 10

Does Not Bother me   Bothers me Very Much

Fatigue During the Day

0 1 2 3 4 5 6 7 8 9 10

Never   Sometimes   Always

Mood

0 1 2 3 4 5 6 7 8 9 10

Cheerful&Calm   Depressed or Anxious

Exercise

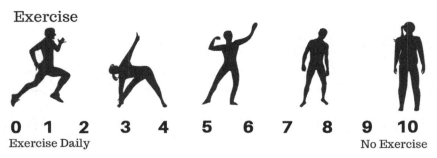

0 1 2 3 4 5 6 7 8 9 10

Exercise Daily   No Exercise

Drugs/Medication

QTY		DESCRIPTION
AM	PM	

Vitamins/Supplements

QTY		DESCRIPTION
AM	PM	

N O T E S

Month: _____ **Day:** Mon Tue Wed Thu Fri Sat Sun

Overall Level of Pain

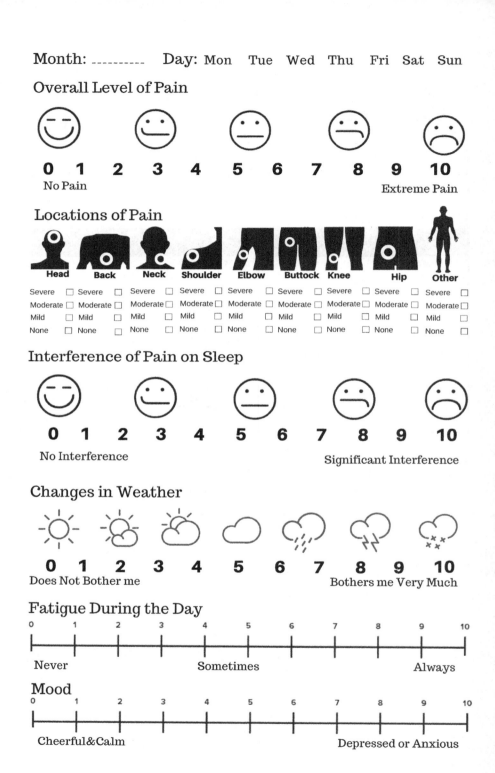

0 1 2 3 4 5 6 7 8 9 10

No Pain   Extreme Pain

Locations of Pain

Head   Back   Neck   Shoulder   Elbow   Buttock   Knee   Hip   Other

	Head	Back	Neck	Shoulder	Elbow	Buttock	Knee	Hip	Other
Severe	☐	☐	☐	☐	☐	☐	☐	☐	☐
Moderate	☐	☐	☐	☐	☐	☐	☐	☐	☐
Mild	☐	☐	☐	☐	☐	☐	☐	☐	☐
None	☐	☐	☐	☐	☐	☐	☐	☐	☐

Interference of Pain on Sleep

0 1 2 3 4 5 6 7 8 9 10

No Interference   Significant Interference

Changes in Weather

0 1 2 3 4 5 6 7 8 9 10

Does Not Bother me   Bothers me Very Much

Fatigue During the Day

0 1 2 3 4 5 6 7 8 9 10

Never   Sometimes   Always

Mood

0 1 2 3 4 5 6 7 8 9 10

Cheerful&Calm   Depressed or Anxious

Exercise

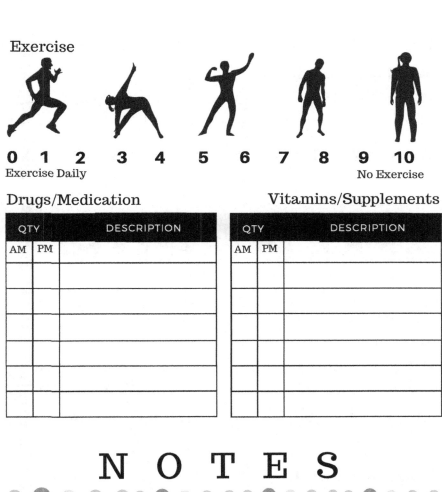

0   1   2   3   4   5   6   7   8   9   10

Exercise Daily   No Exercise

Drugs/Medication

QTY		DESCRIPTION
AM	PM	

Vitamins/Supplements

QTY		DESCRIPTION
AM	PM	

N O T E S

Month: _____ **Day:** Mon   Tue   Wed   Thu   Fri   Sat   Sun

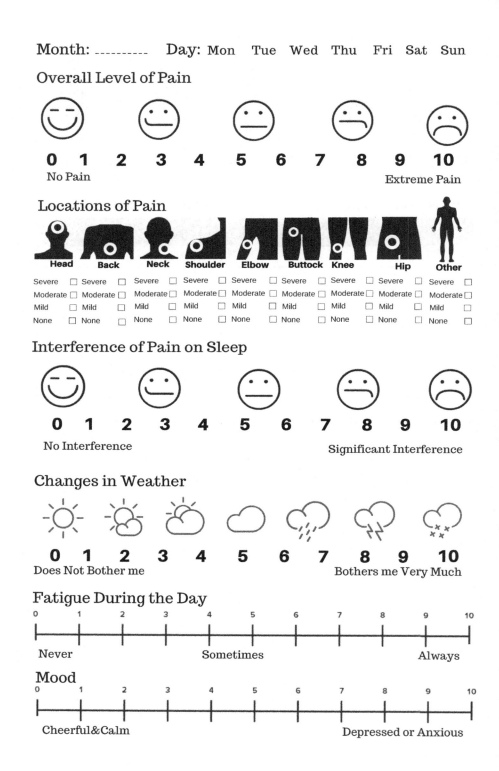

Overall Level of Pain

0 1 2 3 4 5 6 7 8 9 10

No Pain   Extreme Pain

Locations of Pain

Head   Back   Neck   Shoulder   Elbow   Buttock   Knee   Hip   Other

	Head	Back	Neck	Shoulder	Elbow	Buttock	Knee	Hip	Other
Severe	☐	☐	☐	☐	☐	☐	☐	☐	☐
Moderate	☐	☐	☐	☐	☐	☐	☐	☐	☐
Mild	☐	☐	☐	☐	☐	☐	☐	☐	☐
None	☐	☐	☐	☐	☐	☐	☐	☐	☐

Interference of Pain on Sleep

0 1 2 3 4 5 6 7 8 9 10

No Interference   Significant Interference

Changes in Weather

0 1 2 3 4 5 6 7 8 9 10

Does Not Bother me   Bothers me Very Much

Fatigue During the Day

0 1 2 3 4 5 6 7 8 9 10

Never   Sometimes   Always

Mood

0 1 2 3 4 5 6 7 8 9 10

Cheerful&Calm   Depressed or Anxious

Exercise

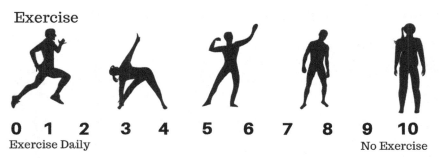

0   1   2   3   4   5   6   7   8   9   10

Exercise Daily   No Exercise

Drugs/Medication

QTY		DESCRIPTION
AM	PM	

Vitamins/Supplements

QTY		DESCRIPTION
AM	PM	

N O T E S

Month: ---------- **Day:** Mon Tue Wed Thu Fri Sat Sun

Overall Level of Pain

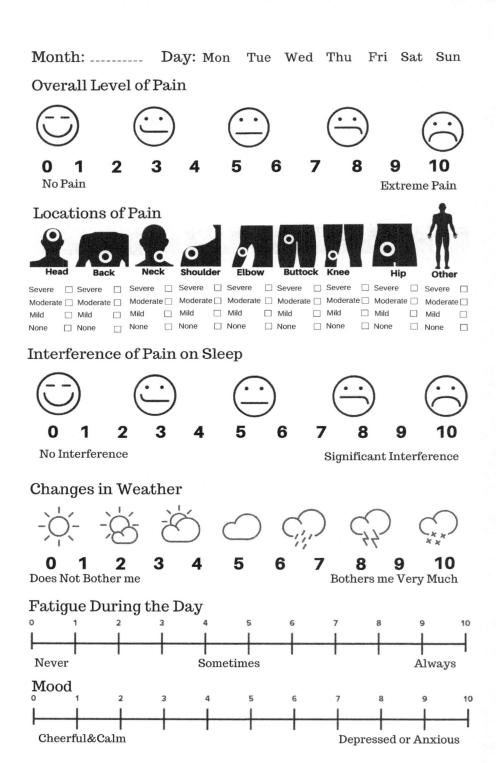

0 1 2 3 4 5 6 7 8 9 10

No Pain   Extreme Pain

Locations of Pain

Head	Back	Neck	Shoulder	Elbow	Buttock	Knee	Hip	Other
Severe ☐	Severe ☐	Severe ☐	Severe ☐	Severe ☐	Severe ☐	Severe ☐	Severe ☐	Severe ☐
Moderate ☐	Moderate ☐	Moderate ☐	Moderate ☐	Moderate ☐	Moderate ☐	Moderate ☐	Moderate ☐	Moderate ☐
Mild ☐	Mild ☐	Mild ☐	Mild ☐	Mild ☐	Mild ☐	Mild ☐	Mild ☐	Mild ☐
None ☐	None ☐	None ☐	None ☐	None ☐	None ☐	None ☐	None ☐	None ☐

Interference of Pain on Sleep

0 1 2 3 4 5 6 7 8 9 10

No Interference   Significant Interference

Changes in Weather

0 1 2 3 4 5 6 7 8 9 10

Does Not Bother me   Bothers me Very Much

Fatigue During the Day

0   1   2   3   4   5   6   7   8   9   10

Never   Sometimes   Always

Mood

0   1   2   3   4   5   6   7   8   9   10

Cheerful&Calm   Depressed or Anxious

Exercise

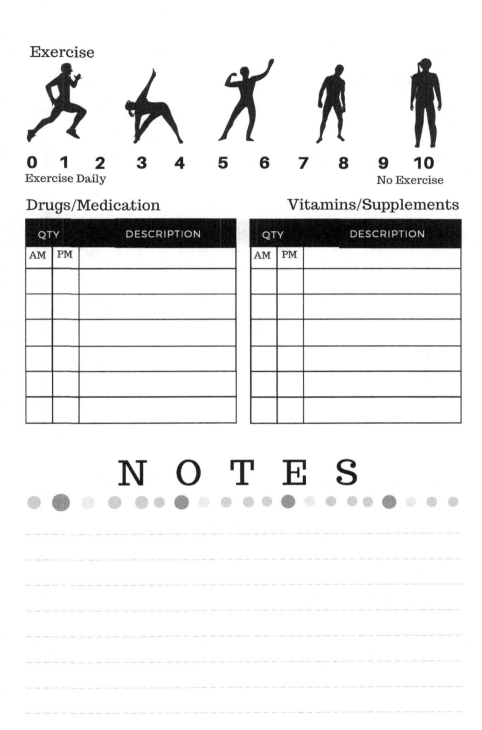

0   1   2   3   4   5   6   7   8   9   10

Exercise Daily   No Exercise

Drugs/Medication

QTY		DESCRIPTION
AM	PM	

Vitamins/Supplements

QTY		DESCRIPTION
AM	PM	

N O T E S

Month: _____ Day: Mon Tue Wed Thu Fri Sat Sun

Overall Level of Pain

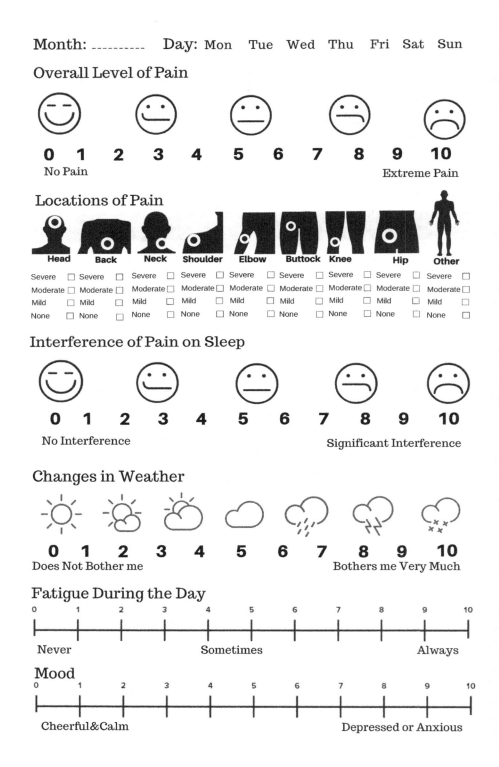

0 1 2 3 4 5 6 7 8 9 10

No Pain   Extreme Pain

Locations of Pain

	Head	Back	Neck	Shoulder	Elbow	Buttock	Knee	Hip	Other
Severe	☐	☐	☐	☐	☐	☐	☐	☐	☐
Moderate	☐	☐	☐	☐	☐	☐	☐	☐	☐
Mild	☐	☐	☐	☐	☐	☐	☐	☐	☐
None	☐	☐	☐	☐	☐	☐	☐	☐	☐

Interference of Pain on Sleep

0 1 2 3 4 5 6 7 8 9 10

No Interference   Significant Interference

Changes in Weather

0 1 2 3 4 5 6 7 8 9 10

Does Not Bother me   Bothers me Very Much

Fatigue During the Day

0   1   2   3   4   5   6   7   8   9   10

Never   Sometimes   Always

Mood

0   1   2   3   4   5   6   7   8   9   10

Cheerful&Calm   Depressed or Anxious

Exercise

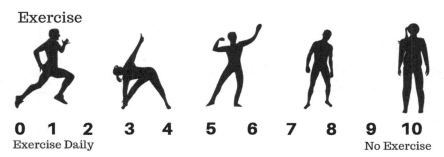

0   1   2   3   4   5   6   7   8   9   10

Exercise Daily   No Exercise

Drugs/Medication

QTY		DESCRIPTION
AM	PM	

Vitamins/Supplements

QTY		DESCRIPTION
AM	PM	

N O T E S

Month: .... Day: Mon Tue Wed Thu Fri Sat Sun

Overall Level of Pain

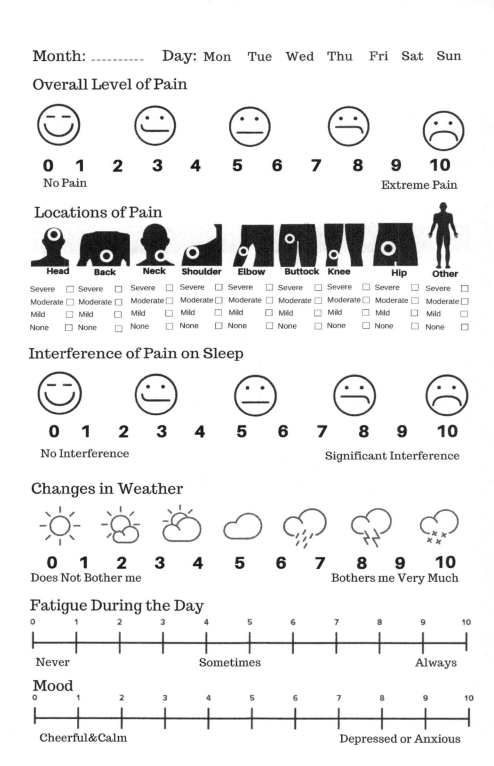

0 1 2 3 4 5 6 7 8 9 10

No Pain   Extreme Pain

Locations of Pain

Head	Back	Neck	Shoulder	Elbow	Buttock	Knee	Hip	Other
Severe ☐	Severe ☐	Severe ☐	Severe ☐	Severe ☐	Severe ☐	Severe ☐	Severe ☐	Severe ☐
Moderate ☐	Moderate ☐	Moderate ☐	Moderate ☐	Moderate ☐	Moderate ☐	Moderate ☐	Moderate ☐	Moderate ☐
Mild ☐	Mild ☐	Mild ☐	Mild ☐	Mild ☐	Mild ☐	Mild ☐	Mild ☐	Mild ☐
None ☐	None ☐	None ☐	None ☐	None ☐	None ☐	None ☐	None ☐	None ☐

Interference of Pain on Sleep

0 1 2 3 4 5 6 7 8 9 10

No Interference   Significant Interference

Changes in Weather

0 1 2 3 4 5 6 7 8 9 10

Does Not Bother me   Bothers me Very Much

Fatigue During the Day

0   1   2   3   4   5   6   7   8   9   10

Never   Sometimes   Always

Mood

0   1   2   3   4   5   6   7   8   9   10

Cheerful&Calm   Depressed or Anxious

Exercise

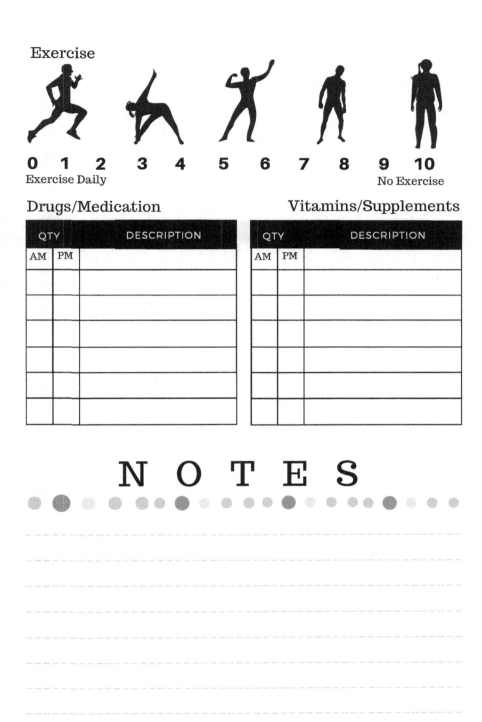

0   1   2   3   4   5   6   7   8   9   10

Exercise Daily   No Exercise

Drugs/Medication

QTY		DESCRIPTION
AM	PM	

Vitamins/Supplements

QTY		DESCRIPTION
AM	PM	

N O T E S

Month: .... **Day:** Mon   Tue   Wed   Thu   Fri   Sat   Sun

Overall Level of Pain

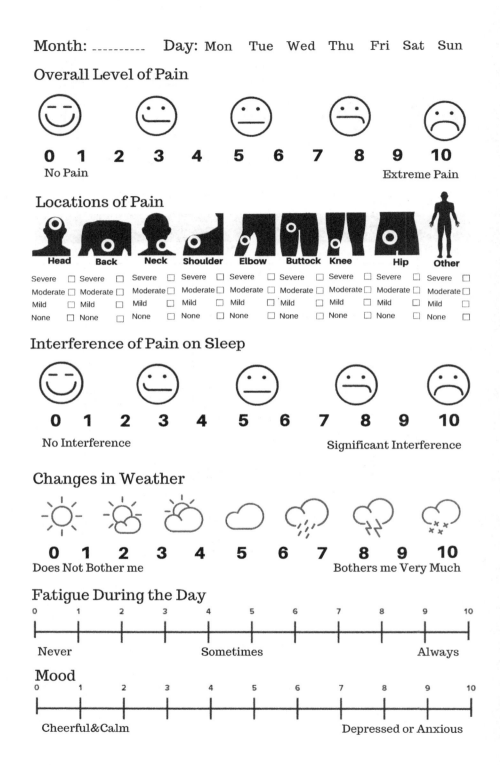

0   1   2   3   4   5   6   7   8   9   10

No Pain   Extreme Pain

Locations of Pain

	Head	Back	Neck	Shoulder	Elbow	Buttock	Knee	Hip	Other
Severe	☐	☐	☐	☐	☐	☐	☐	☐	☐
Moderate	☐	☐	☐	☐	☐	☐	☐	☐	☐
Mild	☐	☐	☐	☐	☐	☐	☐	☐	☐
None	☐	☐	☐	☐	☐	☐	☐	☐	☐

Interference of Pain on Sleep

0   1   2   3   4   5   6   7   8   9   10

No Interference   Significant Interference

Changes in Weather

0   1   2   3   4   5   6   7   8   9   10

Does Not Bother me   Bothers me Very Much

Fatigue During the Day

0   1   2   3   4   5   6   7   8   9   10

Never   Sometimes   Always

Mood

0   1   2   3   4   5   6   7   8   9   10

Cheerful&Calm   Depressed or Anxious

Exercise

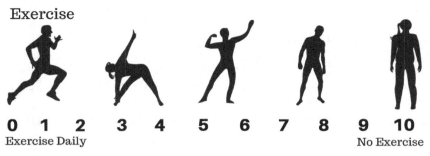

0   1   2   3   4   5   6   7   8   9   10

Exercise Daily   No Exercise

Drugs/Medication

QTY		DESCRIPTION
AM	PM	

Vitamins/Supplements

QTY		DESCRIPTION
AM	PM	

N O T E S

Month: ---------- **Day:** Mon   Tue   Wed   Thu   Fri   Sat   Sun

Overall Level of Pain

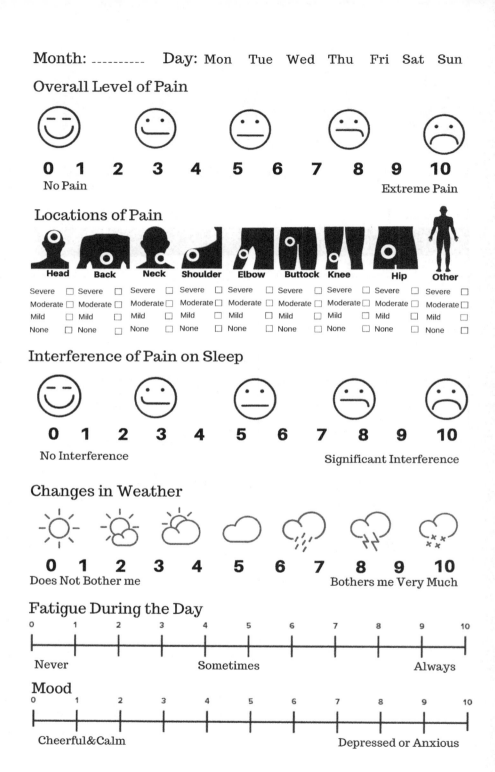

0 1 2 3 4 5 6 7 8 9 10

No Pain   Extreme Pain

Locations of Pain

	Head	Back	Neck	Shoulder	Elbow	Buttock	Knee	Hip	Other
Severe	☐	☐	☐	☐	☐	☐	☐	☐	☐
Moderate	☐	☐	☐	☐	☐	☐	☐	☐	☐
Mild	☐	☐	☐	☐	☐	☐	☐	☐	☐
None	☐	☐	☐	☐	☐	☐	☐	☐	☐

Interference of Pain on Sleep

0 1 2 3 4 5 6 7 8 9 10

No Interference   Significant Interference

Changes in Weather

0 1 2 3 4 5 6 7 8 9 10

Does Not Bother me   Bothers me Very Much

Fatigue During the Day

0 1 2 3 4 5 6 7 8 9 10

Never   Sometimes   Always

Mood

0 1 2 3 4 5 6 7 8 9 10

Cheerful&Calm   Depressed or Anxious

Exercise

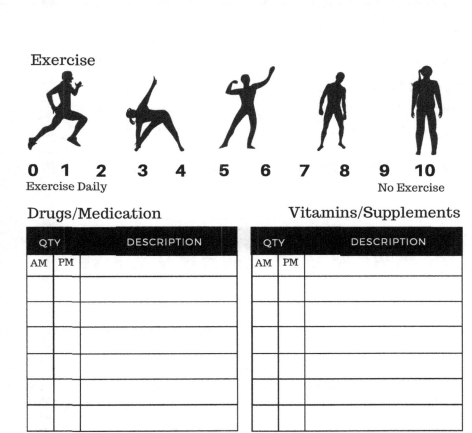

0 1 2   3   4   5   6   7   8   9 10

Exercise Daily   No Exercise

Drugs/Medication

QTY		DESCRIPTION
AM	PM	

Vitamins/Supplements

QTY		DESCRIPTION
AM	PM	

N O T E S

Month: ---------- **Day:** Mon   Tue   Wed   Thu   Fri   Sat   Sun

Overall Level of Pain

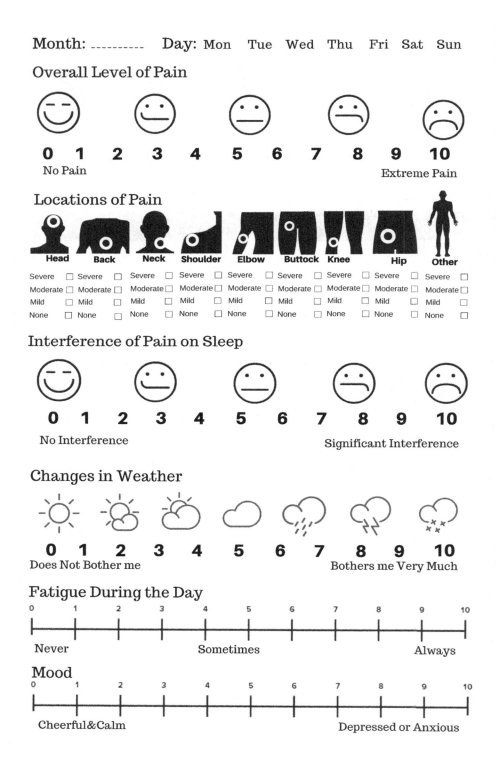

0   1   2   3   4   5   6   7   8   9   10

No Pain   Extreme Pain

Locations of Pain

	Head	Back	Neck	Shoulder	Elbow	Buttock	Knee	Hip	Other
Severe	☐	☐	☐	☐	☐	☐	☐	☐	☐
Moderate	☐	☐	☐	☐	☐	☐	☐	☐	☐
Mild	☐	☐	☐	☐	☐	☐	☐	☐	☐
None	☐	☐	☐	☐	☐	☐	☐	☐	☐

Interference of Pain on Sleep

0   1   2   3   4   5   6   7   8   9   10

No Interference   Significant Interference

Changes in Weather

0   1   2   3   4   5   6   7   8   9   10

Does Not Bother me   Bothers me Very Much

Fatigue During the Day

0   1   2   3   4   5   6   7   8   9   10

Never   Sometimes   Always

Mood

0   1   2   3   4   5   6   7   8   9   10

Cheerful&Calm   Depressed or Anxious

Exercise

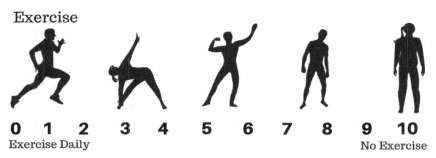

| 0 | 1 | 2 | 3 | 4 | 5 | 6 | 7 | 8 | 9 | 10 |

Exercise Daily   No Exercise

Drugs/Medication

QTY		DESCRIPTION
AM	PM	

Vitamins/Supplements

QTY		DESCRIPTION
AM	PM	

N O T E S

Month: ---------- **Day:** Mon Tue Wed Thu Fri Sat Sun

Overall Level of Pain

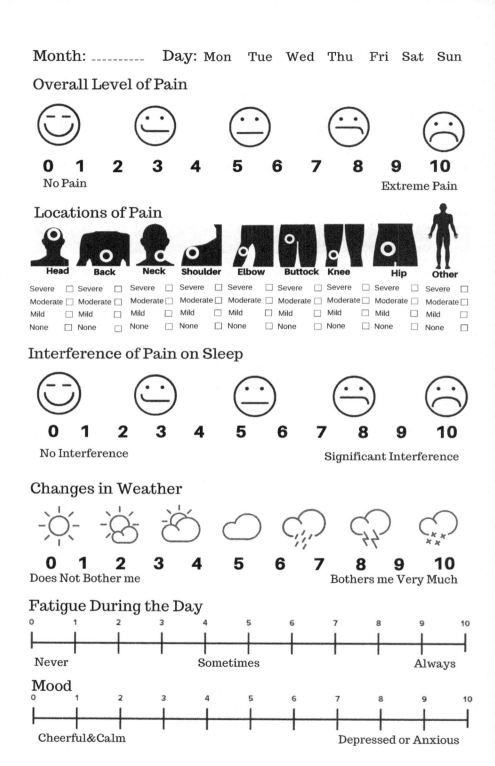

0 1 2 3 4 5 6 7 8 9 10

No Pain   Extreme Pain

Locations of Pain

	Head	Back	Neck	Shoulder	Elbow	Buttock	Knee	Hip	Other
Severe	☐	Severe ☐	Severe ☐	Severe ☐	Severe ☐	Severe ☐	Severe ☐	Severe ☐	Severe ☐
Moderate	☐	Moderate ☐	Moderate ☐	Moderate ☐	Moderate ☐	Moderate ☐	Moderate ☐	Moderate ☐	Moderate ☐
Mild	☐	Mild ☐	Mild ☐	Mild ☐	Mild ☐	Mild ☐	Mild ☐	Mild ☐	Mild ☐
None	☐	None ☐	None ☐	None ☐	None ☐	None ☐	None ☐	None ☐	None ☐

Interference of Pain on Sleep

0 1 2 3 4 5 6 7 8 9 10

No Interference   Significant Interference

Changes in Weather

0 1 2 3 4 5 6 7 8 9 10

Does Not Bother me   Bothers me Very Much

Fatigue During the Day

0   1   2   3   4   5   6   7   8   9   10

Never   Sometimes   Always

Mood

0   1   2   3   4   5   6   7   8   9   10

Cheerful&Calm   Depressed or Anxious

Exercise

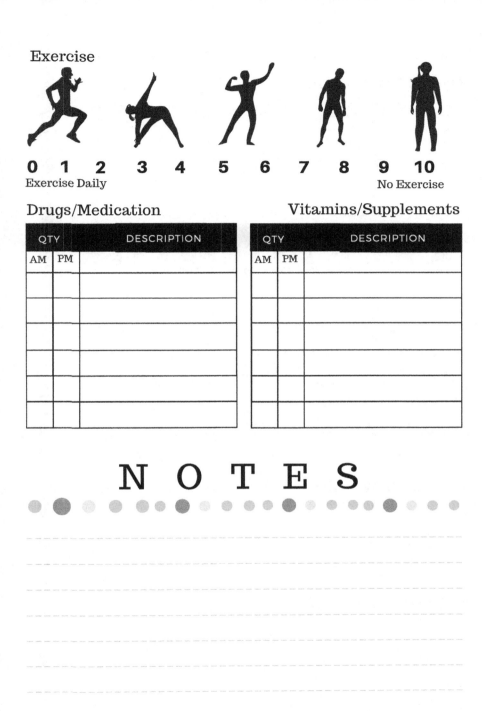

0 1 2 3 4 5 6 7 8 9 10

Exercise Daily   No Exercise

Drugs/Medication

QTY		DESCRIPTION
AM	PM	

Vitamins/Supplements

QTY		DESCRIPTION
AM	PM	

N O T E S

Month: ---------- **Day:** Mon Tue Wed Thu Fri Sat Sun

Overall Level of Pain

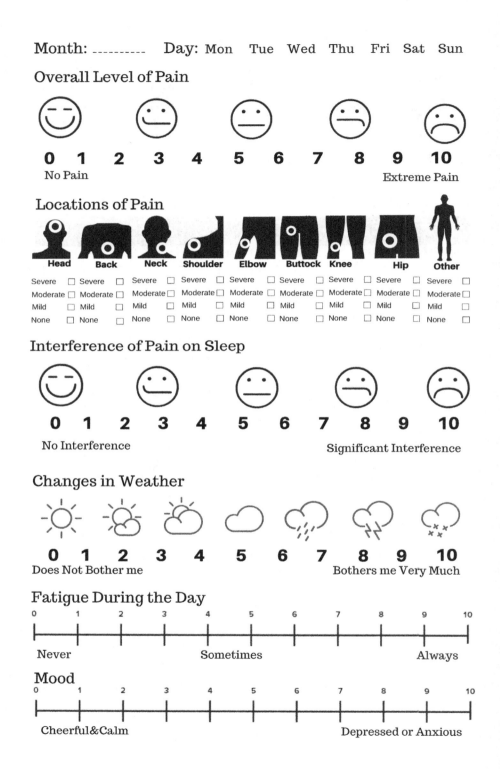

```
0   1   2   3   4   5   6   7   8   9   10
```
No Pain   Extreme Pain

Locations of Pain

	Head	Back	Neck	Shoulder	Elbow	Buttock	Knee	Hip	Other
Severe	☐	☐	☐	☐	☐	☐	☐	☐	☐
Moderate	☐	☐	☐	☐	☐	☐	☐	☐	☐
Mild	☐	☐	☐	☐	☐	☐	☐	☐	☐
None	☐	☐	☐	☐	☐	☐	☐	☐	☐

Interference of Pain on Sleep

```
0   1   2   3   4   5   6   7   8   9   10
```
No Interference   Significant Interference

Changes in Weather

```
0   1   2   3   4   5   6   7   8   9   10
```
Does Not Bother me   Bothers me Very Much

Fatigue During the Day

```
0    1    2    3    4    5    6    7    8    9    10
```
Never   Sometimes   Always

Mood

```
0    1    2    3    4    5    6    7    8    9    10
```
Cheerful&Calm   Depressed or Anxious

Exercise

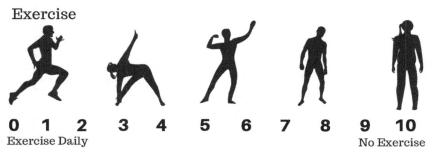

0 1 2 3 4 5 6 7 8 9 10

Exercise Daily   No Exercise

Drugs/Medication

QTY		DESCRIPTION
AM	PM	

Vitamins/Supplements

QTY		DESCRIPTION
AM	PM	

N O T E S

Month: ---------- Day: Mon Tue Wed Thu Fri Sat Sun

Overall Level of Pain

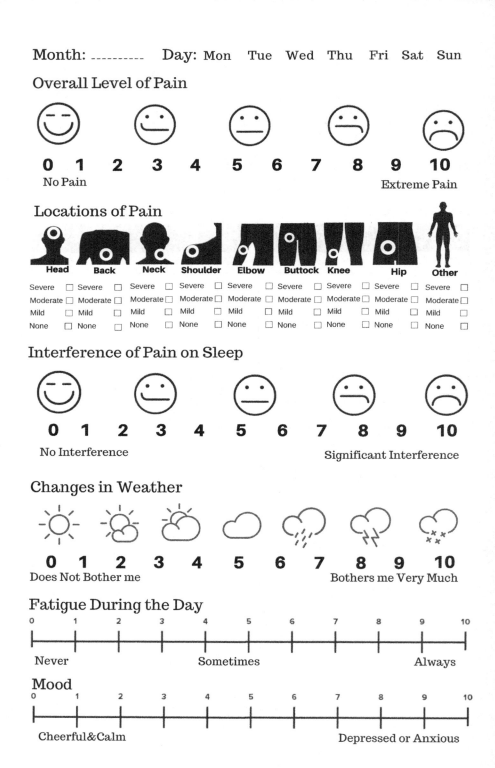

0 1 2 3 4 5 6 7 8 9 10

No Pain   Extreme Pain

Locations of Pain

	Head	Back	Neck	Shoulder	Elbow	Buttock	Knee	Hip	Other
Severe	☐	Severe ☐	Severe ☐	Severe ☐	Severe ☐	Severe ☐	Severe ☐	Severe ☐	Severe ☐
Moderate	☐	Moderate ☐	Moderate ☐	Moderate ☐	Moderate ☐	Moderate ☐	Moderate ☐	Moderate ☐	Moderate ☐
Mild	☐	Mild ☐	Mild ☐	Mild ☐	Mild ☐	Mild ☐	Mild ☐	Mild ☐	Mild ☐
None	☐	None ☐	None ☐	None ☐	None ☐	None ☐	None ☐	None ☐	None ☐

Interference of Pain on Sleep

0 1 2 3 4 5 6 7 8 9 10

No Interference   Significant Interference

Changes in Weather

0 1 2 3 4 5 6 7 8 9 10

Does Not Bother me   Bothers me Very Much

Fatigue During the Day

0 1 2 3 4 5 6 7 8 9 10

Never   Sometimes   Always

Mood

0 1 2 3 4 5 6 7 8 9 10

Cheerful&Calm   Depressed or Anxious

Exercise

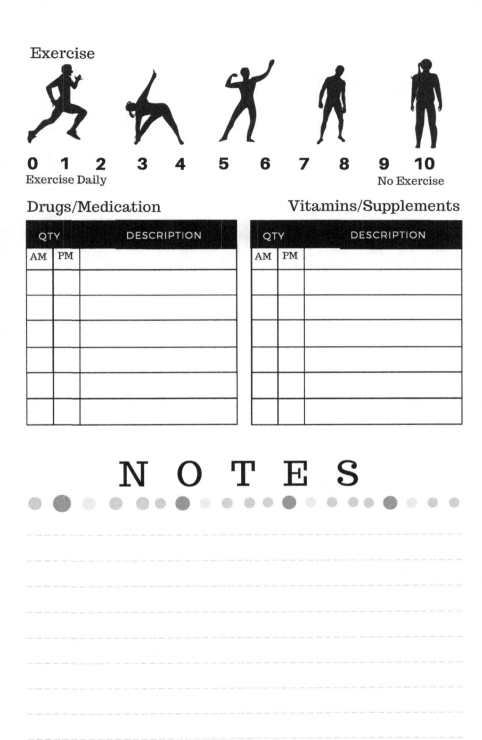

0　1　2　3　4　5　6　7　8　9　10

Exercise Daily　　　　　　　　　　　　No Exercise

Drugs/Medication

QTY		DESCRIPTION
AM	PM	

Vitamins/Supplements

QTY		DESCRIPTION
AM	PM	

N O T E S

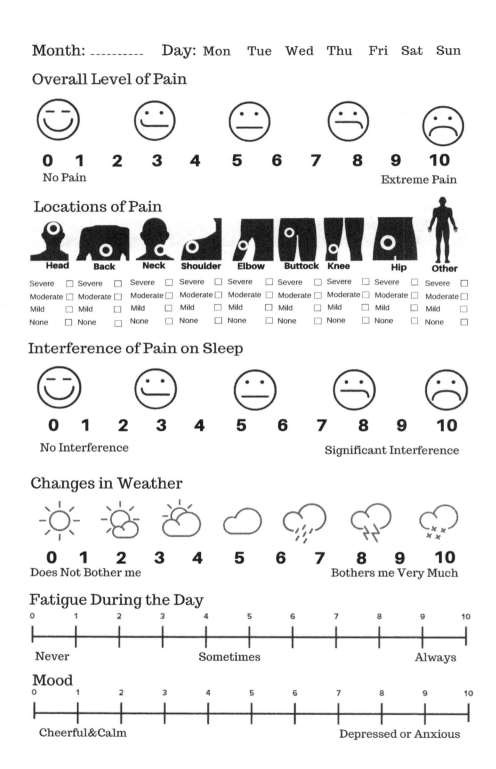

Month: ---------- Day: Mon Tue Wed Thu Fri Sat Sun

Overall Level of Pain

0   1   2   3   4   5   6   7   8   9   10

No Pain   Extreme Pain

Locations of Pain

Head	Back	Neck	Shoulder	Elbow	Buttock	Knee	Hip	Other
Severe ☐	Severe ☐	Severe ☐	Severe ☐	Severe ☐	Severe ☐	Severe ☐	Severe ☐	Severe ☐
Moderate ☐	Moderate ☐	Moderate ☐	Moderate ☐	Moderate ☐	Moderate ☐	Moderate ☐	Moderate ☐	Moderate ☐
Mild ☐	Mild ☐	Mild ☐	Mild ☐	Mild ☐	Mild ☐	Mild ☐	Mild ☐	Mild ☐
None ☐	None ☐	None ☐	None ☐	None ☐	None ☐	None ☐	None ☐	None ☐

Interference of Pain on Sleep

0   1   2   3   4   5   6   7   8   9   10

No Interference   Significant Interference

Changes in Weather

0   1   2   3   4   5   6   7   8   9   10

Does Not Bother me   Bothers me Very Much

Fatigue During the Day

0   1   2   3   4   5   6   7   8   9   10

Never   Sometimes   Always

Mood

0   1   2   3   4   5   6   7   8   9   10

Cheerful&Calm   Depressed or Anxious

Exercise

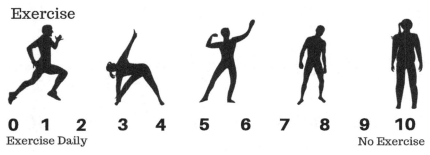

0   1   2   3   4   5   6   7   8   9   10

Exercise Daily   No Exercise

Drugs/Medication

QTY		DESCRIPTION
AM	PM	

Vitamins/Supplements

QTY		DESCRIPTION
AM	PM	

N O T E S

Month: _____ **Day:** Mon Tue Wed Thu Fri Sat Sun

Overall Level of Pain

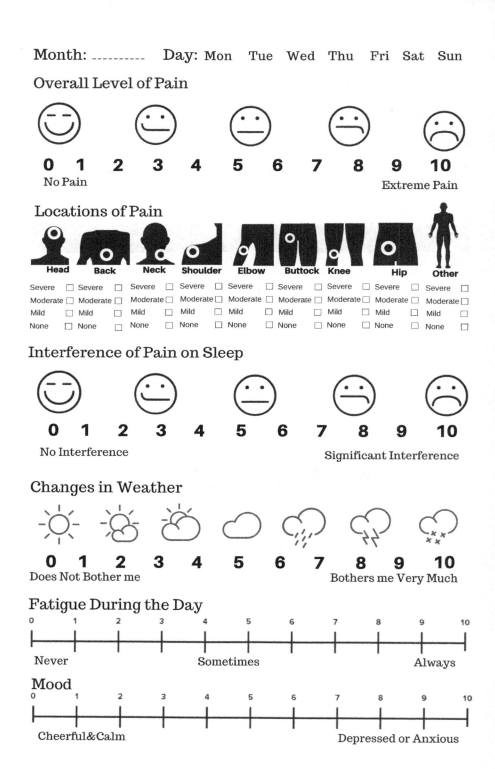

0   1   2   3   4   5   6   7   8   9   10

No Pain   Extreme Pain

Locations of Pain

Head **Back** **Neck** **Shoulder** **Elbow** **Buttock** **Knee** **Hip** **Other**

	Head	Back	Neck	Shoulder	Elbow	Buttock	Knee	Hip	Other
Severe	☐	☐	☐	☐	☐	☐	☐	☐	☐
Moderate	☐	☐	☐	☐	☐	☐	☐	☐	☐
Mild	☐	☐	☐	☐	☐	☐	☐	☐	☐
None	☐	☐	☐	☐	☐	☐	☐	☐	☐

Interference of Pain on Sleep

0   1   2   3   4   5   6   7   8   9   10

No Interference   Significant Interference

Changes in Weather

0   1   2   3   4   5   6   7   8   9   10

Does Not Bother me   Bothers me Very Much

Fatigue During the Day

0   1   2   3   4   5   6   7   8   9   10

Never   Sometimes   Always

Mood

0   1   2   3   4   5   6   7   8   9   10

Cheerful&Calm   Depressed or Anxious

Exercise

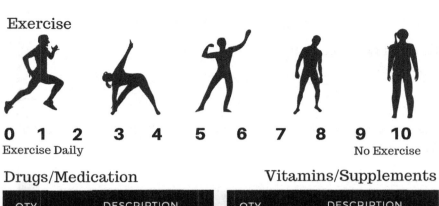

0 1 2 3 4 5 6 7 8 9 10

Exercise Daily   No Exercise

Drugs/Medication

QTY		DESCRIPTION
AM	PM	

Vitamins/Supplements

QTY		DESCRIPTION
AM	PM	

N O T E S

Month: _____ Day: Mon Tue Wed Thu Fri Sat Sun

Overall Level of Pain

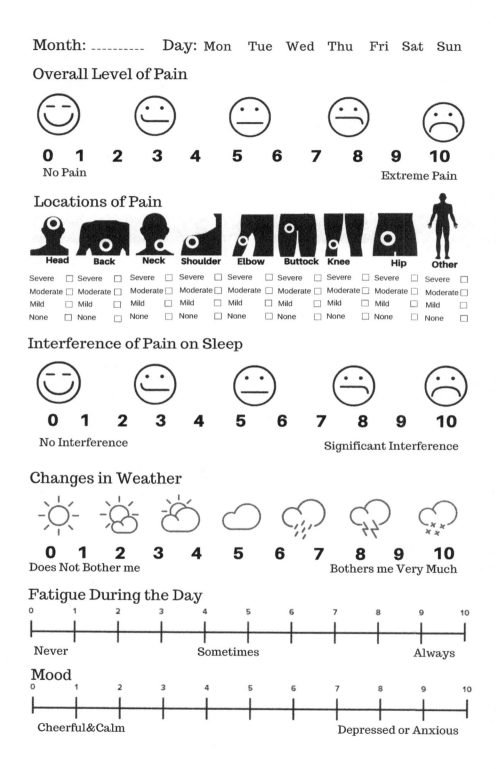

0   1   2   3   4   5   6   7   8   9   10

No Pain   Extreme Pain

Locations of Pain

	Head	Back	Neck	Shoulder	Elbow	Buttock	Knee	Hip	Other
Severe	☐	☐	☐	☐	☐	☐	☐	☐	☐
Moderate	☐	☐	☐	☐	☐	☐	☐	☐	☐
Mild	☐	☐	☐	☐	☐	☐	☐	☐	☐
None	☐	☐	☐	☐	☐	☐	☐	☐	☐

Interference of Pain on Sleep

0   1   2   3   4   5   6   7   8   9   10

No Interference   Significant Interference

Changes in Weather

0   1   2   3   4   5   6   7   8   9   10

Does Not Bother me   Bothers me Very Much

Fatigue During the Day

0   1   2   3   4   5   6   7   8   9   10

Never   Sometimes   Always

Mood

0   1   2   3   4   5   6   7   8   9   10

Cheerful&Calm   Depressed or Anxious

Exercise

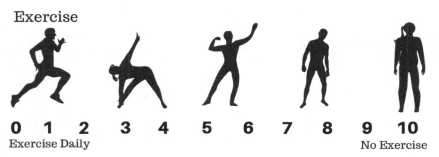

0 1 2 3 4 5 6 7 8 9 10

Exercise Daily   No Exercise

Drugs/Medication

QTY		DESCRIPTION
AM	PM	

Vitamins/Supplements

QTY		DESCRIPTION
AM	PM	

N O T E S

Month: ---------- Day: Mon Tue Wed Thu Fri Sat Sun

Overall Level of Pain

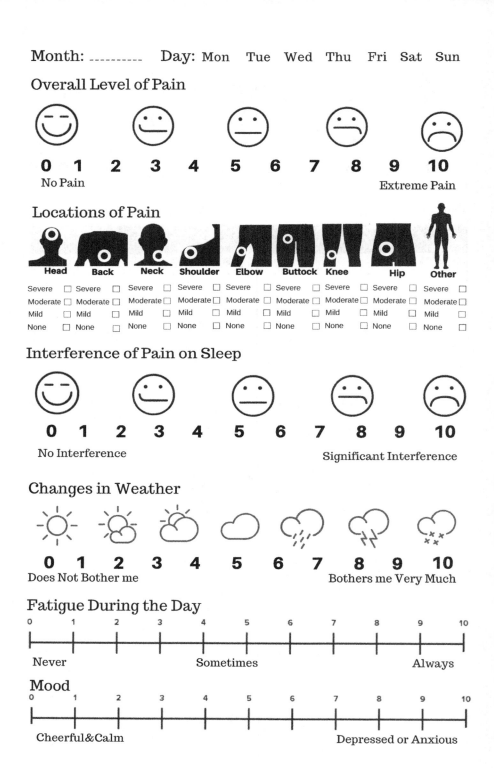

0 1 2 3 4 5 6 7 8 9 10

No Pain   Extreme Pain

Locations of Pain

	Head	Back	Neck	Shoulder	Elbow	Buttock	Knee	Hip	Other
Severe	☐	☐	☐	☐	☐	☐	☐	☐	☐
Moderate	☐	☐	☐	☐	☐	☐	☐	☐	☐
Mild	☐	☐	☐	☐	☐	☐	☐	☐	☐
None	☐	☐	☐	☐	☐	☐	☐	☐	☐

Interference of Pain on Sleep

0 1 2 3 4 5 6 7 8 9 10

No Interference   Significant Interference

Changes in Weather

0 1 2 3 4 5 6 7 8 9 10

Does Not Bother me   Bothers me Very Much

Fatigue During the Day

0 1 2 3 4 5 6 7 8 9 10

Never   Sometimes   Always

Mood

0 1 2 3 4 5 6 7 8 9 10

Cheerful&Calm   Depressed or Anxious

Exercise

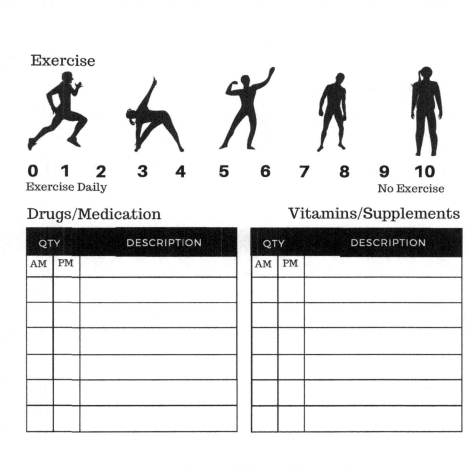

0 1 2   3 4   5   6   7   8   9 10

Exercise Daily   No Exercise

Drugs/Medication

QTY		DESCRIPTION
AM	PM	

Vitamins/Supplements

QTY		DESCRIPTION
AM	PM	

N O T E S

Month: ---------- **Day:** Mon Tue Wed Thu Fri Sat Sun

Overall Level of Pain

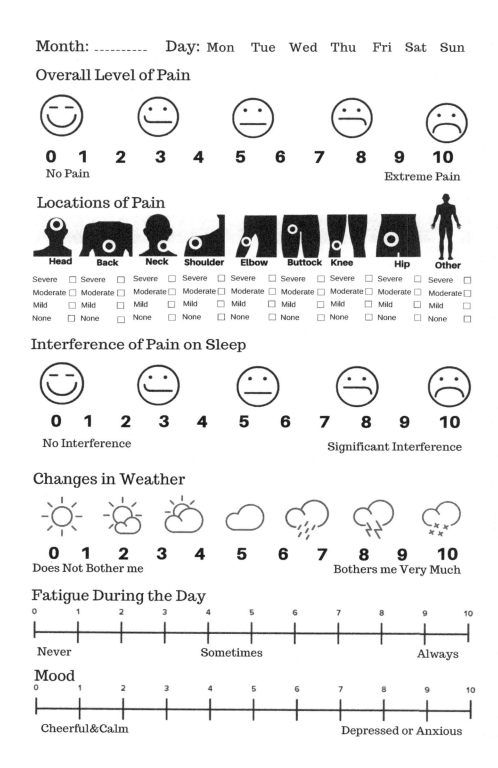

0 1 2 3 4 5 6 7 8 9 10

No Pain   Extreme Pain

Locations of Pain

	Head	Back	Neck	Shoulder	Elbow	Buttock	Knee	Hip	Other
Severe	☐	☐	☐	☐	☐	☐	☐	☐	☐
Moderate	☐	☐	☐	☐	☐	☐	☐	☐	☐
Mild	☐	☐	☐	☐	☐	☐	☐	☐	☐
None	☐	☐	☐	☐	☐	☐	☐	☐	☐

Interference of Pain on Sleep

0 1 2 3 4 5 6 7 8 9 10

No Interference   Significant Interference

Changes in Weather

0 1 2 3 4 5 6 7 8 9 10

Does Not Bother me   Bothers me Very Much

Fatigue During the Day

0   1   2   3   4   5   6   7   8   9   10

Never   Sometimes   Always

Mood

0   1   2   3   4   5   6   7   8   9   10

Cheerful&Calm   Depressed or Anxious

Exercise

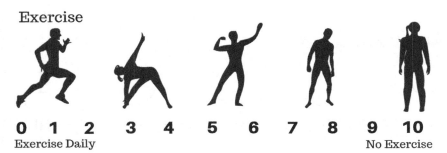

0 1 2   3   4   5   6   7   8   9 10

Exercise Daily   No Exercise

Drugs/Medication

QTY		DESCRIPTION
AM	PM	

Vitamins/Supplements

QTY		DESCRIPTION
AM	PM	

N O T E S

Month: _____ **Day:** Mon Tue Wed Thu Fri Sat Sun

Overall Level of Pain

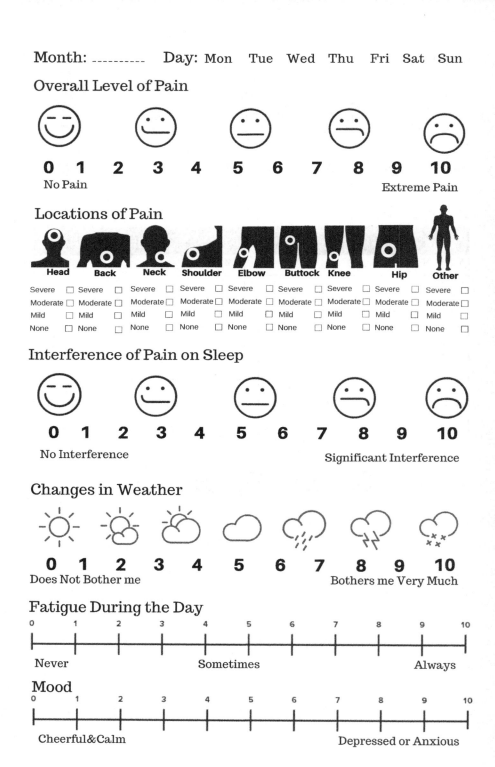

0 1 2 3 4 5 6 7 8 9 10

No Pain   Extreme Pain

Locations of Pain

	Head	Back	Neck	Shoulder	Elbow	Buttock	Knee	Hip	Other
Severe	☐	Severe ☐	Severe ☐	Severe ☐	Severe ☐	Severe ☐	Severe ☐	Severe ☐	Severe ☐
Moderate	☐	Moderate ☐	Moderate ☐	Moderate ☐	Moderate ☐	Moderate ☐	Moderate ☐	Moderate ☐	Moderate ☐
Mild	☐	Mild ☐	Mild ☐	Mild ☐	Mild ☐	Mild ☐	Mild ☐	Mild ☐	Mild ☐
None	☐	None ☐	None ☐	None ☐	None ☐	None ☐	None ☐	None ☐	None ☐

Interference of Pain on Sleep

0 1 2 3 4 5 6 7 8 9 10

No Interference   Significant Interference

Changes in Weather

0 1 2 3 4 5 6 7 8 9 10

Does Not Bother me   Bothers me Very Much

Fatigue During the Day

0   1   2   3   4   5   6   7   8   9   10

Never   Sometimes   Always

Mood

0   1   2   3   4   5   6   7   8   9   10

Cheerful&Calm   Depressed or Anxious

Exercise

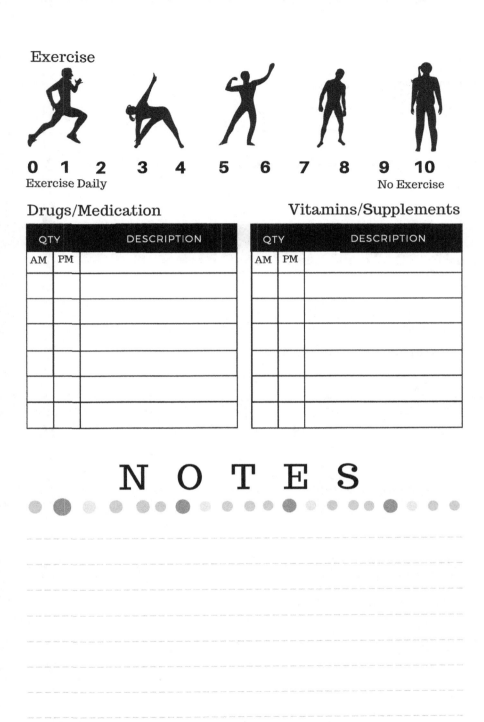

0 1 2   3   4   5   6   7   8   9 10

Exercise Daily   No Exercise

Drugs/Medication

QTY		DESCRIPTION
AM	PM	

Vitamins/Supplements

QTY		DESCRIPTION
AM	PM	

N O T E S

Month: ---------- Day: Mon Tue Wed Thu Fri Sat Sun

Overall Level of Pain

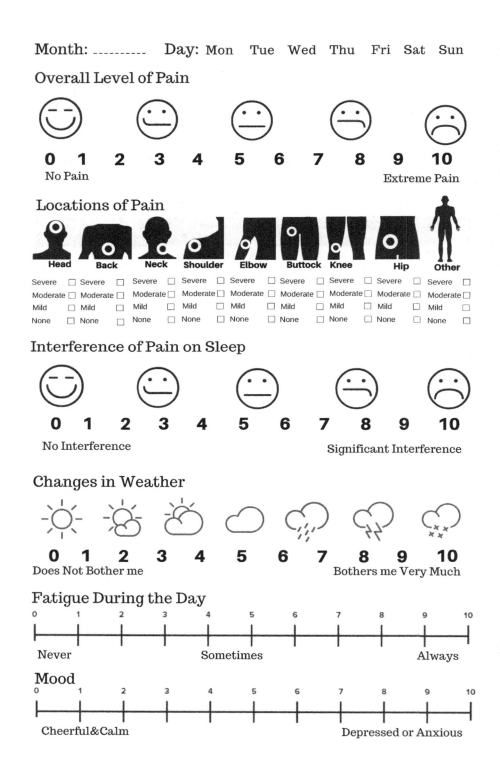

0 1 2 3 4 5 6 7 8 9 10

No Pain   Extreme Pain

Locations of Pain

	Head	Back	Neck	Shoulder	Elbow	Buttock	Knee	Hip	Other
Severe	☐	☐	☐	☐	☐	☐	☐	☐	☐
Moderate	☐	☐	☐	☐	☐	☐	☐	☐	☐
Mild	☐	☐	☐	☐	☐	☐	☐	☐	☐
None	☐	☐	☐	☐	☐	☐	☐	☐	☐

Interference of Pain on Sleep

0 1 2 3 4 5 6 7 8 9 10

No Interference   Significant Interference

Changes in Weather

0 1 2 3 4 5 6 7 8 9 10

Does Not Bother me   Bothers me Very Much

Fatigue During the Day

0   1   2   3   4   5   6   7   8   9   10

Never   Sometimes   Always

Mood

0   1   2   3   4   5   6   7   8   9   10

Cheerful&Calm   Depressed or Anxious

Exercise

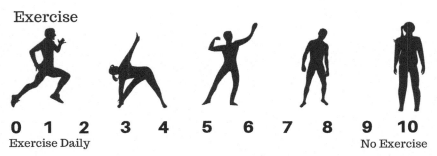

0 1 2   3   4   5   6   7   8   9 10

Exercise Daily   No Exercise

Drugs/Medication

QTY		DESCRIPTION
AM	PM	

Vitamins/Supplements

QTY		DESCRIPTION
AM	PM	

N O T E S

Made in the USA
Coppell, TX
20 April 2022

76844545R00070